Catherine Steven is a former Fleet Street reporter, a writer and medical journalist. She has contributed to the health pages of most national newspapers, women's magazines and specialist journals.

YOUR CHILD SERIES

A series of books containing easy-to-follow, practical advice for the parents of children with a variety of illnesses or conditions.

Each book provides a clear overview of the situation, explaining essential information about the illness or condition and outlining the practical steps parents can take to help understand, support and care for their child, the rest of the family as well as themselves. Guiding parents through the conventional, the complementary and the alternative approaches available, these books cater for children of all ages, ranging from babies to teenagers, and enable the whole family to move forward in a positive way.

Other books in the series:

YOUR CHILD

Diabetes
Practical and Easy-to-Follow Advice

Catherine Steven

ELEMENT

Shaftesbury, Dorset • Boston, Massachusetts
Melbourne, Victoria

© Element Books Limited 1998
Text © Catherine Steven 1998

First published in Great Britain in 1998 by
Element Books Limited
Shaftesbury, Dorset SP7 8BP

Published in the USA in 1998 by
Element Books, Inc.
160 North Washington St, Boston MA 02114

Published in Australia in 1998 by
Element Books and distributed
by Penguin Books Australia Ltd
487 Maroondah Highway, Ringwood,
Victoria 3134

Cover design by Slatter–Anderson
Page design by Roger Lightfoot
Typeset by Bournemouth Colour Press, Parkstone
Printed and bound in Great Britain by Creative Print & Design, Wales

British Library Cataloguing in Publication
data available

Library of Congress-in-Publication Data
Steven, Catherine, 1956–
[Diabetes]
Your child : diabetes / Catherine Steven,
p. cm.
Previously published in 1995 under the title Diabetes
includes bibliographical references and index.
ISBN 1–86204 208–X
1. Diabetes in children—Popular works. I. Title.
RJ420.D5S/4 1998 97 48332
618.92'462—dc21 CIP

ISBN 1 86204 208 X

Contents

Introduction

Insulin-dependent diabetes is an incurable, auto-immune disease which arrives with little or no prior warning. A diagnosis for a young child translates to a lifetime of insulin injections and concerns about their future health. It is one of the fastest-growing, and most common, childhood diseases – one child under the age of five is diagnosed every day in the United Kingdom; in the United States the number of affected young people under the age of 16 has doubled over the past ten years. World-wide there are between 100 and 120 million people with diabetes, although this figure includes both maturity-onset and juvenile-onset diabetes, which are different types of the disease.

Diabetes is a highly stressful condition, with repercussions for every member of the immediate family. There are so many rules to follow, so many medical responsibilities for parents, who must learn to 'treat' their child day in day out by giving injections and supervising blood testing, as well as ensuring their child has the right combinations of food and exercise to stay healthy. For some families this is an overwhelming and extremely difficult regime to follow.

This book looks at the stresses and strains diabetes imposes on the family (in nine cases out of ten diabetes strikes in families where there is no previous history of the disease), and offers guidance to help parents come to terms with the loss of their 'healthy' child. It also contains suggestions for boosting their child's self-esteem, encouraging their body's own natural healing process, and arming them with the confidence to face the future challenges of diabetes which they must eventually confront alone.

Administering insulin is the only life-saving treatment for insulin-dependent diabetes, but complementary therapies can be an enormous help to the condition by keeping stress levels to a minimum, helping to alleviate the anxiety of living with diabetes and boosting the body's own internal healing systems. This book explores soothing techniques such as relaxation, diet, yoga, massage and hypnotherapy, as well as an exciting new method from America. Methods of supporting the body with nutritional therapy and the inclusion of vital trace minerals important for the health of young people with diabetes are also suggested. It explains the role of zinc, chromium and magnesium in your child's diet, and looks at the effectiveness of Eastern medicine, the way Ayurvedic therapies help control blood sugar levels and whether traditional Chinese medicine might be useful. A good, healthy diet is the basis of your child's health and this book offers sensible wholesome advice to support the immune system and encourage optimum health.

Many children with diabetes suffer an emotional crisis in their adolescent years and deny they have the disease, consequently refusing or 'forgetting' to take their insulin. This has potentially devastating consequences and can pave the way for the development of some of the serious complications of diabetes such as heart or kidney disease. By offering them complementary therapies to help ease this chaotic period in their young lives, we may also be throwing them a lifeline for the future.

Although the whole idea of diabetes and injections may seem terrifying to a family with a newly diagnosed child, there is a tremendous amount to be positive about. Positive thinking helps to keep diabetes in perspective and maintain balance. Seventy-five years ago insulin became the first hormone-replacement therapy to really work – by saving lives. Before that children died within a few years of diagnosis, or suffered the trauma of a near-starvation diet, the only 'treatment' available. Today children with diabetes can eat satisfying and wholesome diets not very different from those of their friends, join in virtually all forms of sport and exercise, grow to become healthy, fulfilled adults, and go on to have families of their own. But at every stage of development on the road to adulthood there will be new obstacles to face and overcome as diabetes will remain a constant presence. And at every new stage, extra support may be found from complementary therapies.

Millions of pounds are being spent in the United States, the United Kingdom, Scandinavia and other European centres to establish why some children, and not others, are affected by diabetes. Until an answer is found the only positive way forward is to get on and live with the disease, day by day. Hurdles can be crossed hand in hand with affected children until they reach an age when they are ready to manage the condition alone, with confidence. The experience of living with diabetes will ultimately help them mature into stronger, and possibly more rounded, human beings.

The aim of this book is to provide support on the journey towards a healthy, fulfilling future for every member of the family with diabetes in its midst.

Catherine Steven
July 1997

Note: 'He' and 'she' are used to describe your child in alternate chapters, to avoid the more cumbersome 'he or she'. You may also see the terms 'blood glucose' and 'blood sugars' which, for the purposes of this book, are the same thing. 'Glucose' is the strict medical definition while 'sugars' is a term also in common use.

Chapter One

What is diabetes?

Diabetes is a complex metabolic disorder which develops when insulin-producing cells in the pancreas, a gland behind the stomach, either fail to work properly or are attacked and destroyed by the body's own immune system.

In almost every case there is a genetic predisposition towards the disease – sufferers will have inherited a flawed gene making them susceptible to diabetes. But they will also have been exposed to one or more triggers, such as an environmental toxin or a virus, with the ability to kick-start the condition. Precisely which are the triggers (there are several being investigated) remains a scientific mystery. If the puzzle can be solved then defeating the disease will become a real possibility.

THE IMPORTANCE OF INSULIN

The pancreas is the insulin-producing factory within the body. Cells in the pancreas which stimulate insulin secretion are called beta-cells (sometimes written as ß-cells) and are found in the pancreatic tissue called the islets of Langherans. In most cases of childhood diabetes 70–90 per cent of these beta-cells are already destroyed by the time of diagnosis. By this stage only small amounts of insulin are being produced, and the destruction of these cells continues until the pancreas no longer makes any insulin at all.

Insulin is a key hormone for life, empowered with the vital job of metabolizing food, through the conversion of proteins, fats and carbohydrates in the diet into energy which can be carried in the bloodstream and made accessible to all cells. Our brains and muscles can only accept energy in the form of glucose, and insulin is vital for its production.

Insulin also holds the key to opening the door to the cells, allowing glucose to enter. When no insulin is produced, the glucose from foods we eat is left in the bloodstream, with no access to the right body cells. Sugar or 'glucose' levels continue to rise – unable to reach the parts of the body requiring this energy – and the excess begins to spill out into the urine.

Although the mechanics of the disease are understood, it is still not clear why diabetes affects some children and not others. It is recognized that there is a genetic element, but this is not the whole picture as there are many examples of a single affected child in a family with no previous history of diabetes on either side of the parental line. Indeed, only 10 per cent of affected children have a diabetic parent and, oddly, diabetes frequently affects just one of a pair of identical twins – in two thirds of cases.

Case Study

Kevin was 11 years old when he was diagnosed with diabetes. He and his identical twin brother David are typical boys, on the go all the time. We noticed something was wrong when we flew out of England for a holiday in Florida – on the way Kevin was incredibly thirsty but we thought it was the excitement and the flight.

Over the next few days he was still very thirsty and one night he complained that his stomach hurt, but it was not until we got back to England that we took him to the doctor. At the initial urine test his blood sugar level was something like 25 or 26! He was taken straight to hospital and we stayed there for about four or five days.

Kevin has injected himself from day one and he has been

wonderful about it. But as parents we did wonder why it was Kevin, and not David, or both of them. The one difference between Kevin and his brother was his numerous visits to hospital in previous years. Kevin broke a leg at four and a half, an arm at age ten, which he re-broke nine months later. He had also been in hospital for a hernia operation and had a very nasty accident on his bike. He was scuffed up from head to toe on the left side, and was very upset and shaken by this experience.

Because he is an identical twin we are keeping an eye on David. He has had blood tests which show a slight sign that his pancreas is not working 100 per cent, but apart from that he is fine. Sometimes David wishes he did have diabetes – Kevin goes away on special camps and holidays with a local diabetes group and David is unbelievably envious about this.

However David also does keep an eye out for Kevin and he is a support to him. As a family we all do blood tests so that Kevin does not feel like he is the only one – Kevin knows a lot about his condition and the importance of monitoring his blood glucose levels.

Avril, mother of identical twins Kevin and David, aged 14

Diabetes in ancient times
The ancient Egyptians defined diabetes as 'the passing of too much urine' and used a high-fibre potion of crushed bones, wheat grains, green lead, earth and water to treat the illness. The medicine is described on an Egyptian papyrus dating back to 1500 BC.

The ancient Greeks later named the disease *diabetes*, which means 'to flow through', a very graphic description. The Latin term *mellitus* which means honeyed or sweet, was added later, creating the term *diabetes mellitus*, or honeyed flow, which describes the sweet, sugar-filled urine of a child with diabetes.

■ SYMPTOMS

Children develop the symptoms of diabetes when between 70 and 90 per cent of the insulin-producing cells in the pancreas are destroyed. The key signs of the disease are:

- **The need to pass large amounts of urine frequently.** This is the kidneys' response to high sugar levels in the urine.
- **An unquenchable thirst.** Water is drawn from body cells to flush out the excess glucose in the system resulting in dehydration.
- **Weight loss.** If sugar cannot be converted into energy the body looks for another source and begins to break down the body's fat and protein which releases sugar into the bloodstream, but escalates the problem.
- **Tiredness.** This is the result of having inadequate and unbalanced energy levels.
- **Blurred vision.** High glucose levels can affect the lens of the eye, causing some blurring of vision. Sight returns to normal two or three weeks after insulin treatment has begun.
- **Moodiness.** This is due to the disruption of the body's hormonal system.
- **Itchy genitals and infections**. Your child may be prone to more urinary infections, abscesses or fungal infections such as thrush because of higher than normal levels of glucose in the urine.

Case Study

Anna went into a diabetic coma at the age of 26 months, two days after Christmas. She had been very low for about four months – losing weight and emotionally very up and down. Health professionals had put it down to her age, being a toddler and being fussy about her food. But she was not a vibrant, strong, child and looking back had probably not been well since the time of her birth.

That winter all the family had been ill with flu-type

illnesses, two or three times. It was just over Christmas that Anna began drinking a lot – and on Christmas Day the excessive urination began, with her wetting the bed. The day after Christmas she had had pizza for supper and she seemed alert and fine, but when she woke in the morning she said she felt terrible and collapsed on to the sofa. I took her to the doctor and on 27 December he did a urine test and confirmed it was diabetes. By this time I had more or less figured it out, but it was still shocking. We spent eight days in hospital after which Anna was a changed child – she began eating properly, sleeping properly, she was more comfortable and a lot calmer – it was as if her personality changed.

At first you think thank goodness it is not a catastrophic disease and thank goodness we now know the reasons for her being ill, but then it sinks in that this is for the rest of your life.

Ingrid, mother of Anna, aged five

TYPES OF DIABETES

Type I diabetes

Most children diagnosed with diabetes will be suffering from Type I diabetes, otherwise known as juvenile-onset diabetes. The incidence of Type I diabetes is escalating every year, and scientists are engaged in a global hunt for the cause. Environmental agents such as viruses, toxins and nitrates are all being investigated.

This is the type of diabetes your child will most probably be suffering from, and is a result of immune-system cells attacking the insulin-producing cells in the pancreas. The T-cells of the immune system recognize the islet cells as 'foreign' and produce substances that destroy them. This auto-immune attack starts early in life – in some cases before the age of two or even in the womb .

By the time Type I diabetes is diagnosed most of the vital

insulin-producing cells in the pancreas will have been destroyed. The peak time for diagnosis is around puberty, when growth and sexual hormones (which have anti-insulin actions) surge through the body.

Screening tests available in the United Kingdom and the United States can now reveal those at risk, but they will not be widely offered until a preventative for the disease is found. New research in America is focusing on how to stop diabetes in its tracks by looking at ways to stop the immune response. One new theory suggests that for some time the beta-cells are only injured by this process and not completely killed off until one event – maybe a virus – acts as the final catalyst. If the immune attack can be halted early in the process it is hoped that 'full blown' diabetes can be prevented.

Type II diabetes

This is a quite separate disorder, and the most common form of diabetes. The symptoms are the same, but the mechanisms of the disease are different. Type II diabetes usually affects people who are over 40 and overweight. Inactivity and obesity can, in susceptible people, inhibit the production and effectiveness of insulin. As a result the body develops 'insulin resistance' – the hormone cannot reach the right receptor cells in the body, which leads to a rise in glucose levels in the blood and the development of the symptoms of the disease. For many people diet – the use of foods which actively lower blood glucose such as guar gum bread or the Indian plant karela, exercise and, as a last resort, glucose-lowering tablets are enough to keep the disease stable, but in severe cases insulin treatment is required.

Maturity-onset diabetes in the young

This form of diabetes was recognized only relatively recently, in the 1970s. It can affect young people under the age of 25 and initially may be confused with Type I diabetes. Often defined as hyperglycaemia (high blood sugar levels), it is usually treatable for at least five years without insulin by paying attention to lifestyle. This form of the disease is hereditary but can be well controlled by diet, exercise and possibly the introduction of glucose-lowering tablets.

Ask a naturopath or nutritional therapist for specialist advice and boost the diet with chromium, magnesium and B and E vitamins, which will improve health as well as help to support existing pancreatic function. In some cases the complications of the disease never evolve.

Transient/neonatal diabetes

This is an extremely rare form of diabetes which can occur during the first month of life, lasts more than two weeks, and requires insulin treatment. But it does not necessarily mean a baby will go on to develop diabetes later in life. Continue breast feeding a baby with neonatal diabetes as this will help to support the immune system. Doctors believe that this form of transient diabetes may be a 'pre-diabetic state', and parents are advised to continue monitoring their children for symptoms of diabetes, even if the condition disappears.

Brittle diabetes

This term is used to describe an instability in the disease rather than a form. Children might go through a 'bad patch' with their diabetes, with severe highs and lows in glucose control. This is most likely to happen during adolescence, and most often affects teenage girls. The condition will settle down with maturity and an acceptance of the disease. Parents are best advised to help their children through this stage, in which they may 'deny' their illness, even secretly fail to take their insulin, as they struggle with the concept that diabetes is a life-long condition. Counselling may help.

In summary

Children with diabetes generally have the Type I (insulin-dependent) form, which is a condition for life. There is, however, an enormous amount that parents can do to boost their health and their own internal healing powers. Holistic therapies have the ability to soothe and calm, as well as to strengthen the child in many different areas of life. Good, wholesome nutrition lays the foundation for a healthy life which will fight the complications that can develop in later life. Yoga and meditation, which are explored in later chapters, will help empower even very young children and enable them to put their disorder into perspective, to accept it as part of who they are. Therapies for the mind and body include wonderful energizing aromatherapy and homeopathy, which can be used to help rid the body of toxins which may have triggered the diabetes in the first instance. Complementary therapies help to develop the child's sense of self-worth, and show that life can be lived to the full with diabetes.

COMPLICATIONS OF TYPE I DIABETES

Hypos

Hypoglycaemia – usually called a 'hypo' – is likely to be the most common complication of your child's diabetes on an everyday basis. It is also one of the most serious, with potentially damaging consequences in the long term. When a young child suffers many uncontrolled hypos and subsequent convulsions, the effect on the brain appears to be cumulative.

Hypos happen when your child's blood glucose levels fall too low, which may be caused by too much insulin, missing a meal or snack or active play without eating enough carbohydrate food beforehand. You can check the position by doing a quick blood test; if the levels indicate that blood glucose levels are 3 millimoles per litre of blood or less (3mmol/l) then your child is in the throes of a hypo.

Symptoms of hypos

The symptoms of a hypo are the result of the brain being starved of glucose. In severe cases the brain is unable to function properly, resulting in confusion and coma. Mood swings are a common feature of a childhood hypo.

The most vulnerable group of children are the under 5s, who may not be able to articulate the early warning signals. Research in Ontario, Canada, in the late 1980s suggested that the intellectual abilities of children with diabetes under the age of 4 can be affected by convulsions, which are sometimes associated with hypos, as well as frequent hypos. Dr Brian Frier of the Royal Infirmary, Edinburgh, Scotland, suggests that repeated hypos may affect the developing brain enough to lower IQ levels in the future, a problem called 'cognitive impairment'.

The key to treating a hypo is to identify the specific warning signs. This is a new approach, and the result of studies carried out by the Department of Diabetes at the Royal Infirmary, Edinburgh, and the Departments of Child Life and Health and Psychology at the University of Edinburgh, Scotland.

A research trial involving 100 children aged between 18 months and 16 years recorded the hypo symptoms of each child. It concluded for the first time that children's hypo symptoms differ from those of adults – there was a far stronger emphasis on behavioural problems being important warning signs. Common behavioural problems have been identified as:

- temper tantrums
- tearfulness
- irritability
- mood swings or argumentativeness
- withdrawal

Action: Look for the *particular* early warning signal in your child – and you will be sure to find a recurring 'theme' . It is vital to act swiftly to reverse the hypo at an early stage – the onset of whingeing, crying or irritability.

The first time a hypo happens can be frightening for you and your child, but the good news is that hypos can usually be reversed quickly.

Dr Frier advises:

Pre-school children are very vulnerable to glucose deprivation in the brain. It is difficult for a child to articulate his symptoms so carers have to be able to recognize the symptoms of a hypo. Under the age of six they cannot give good descriptions although they might say 'I have a sore tummy' or feel unwell.

A notable sign is behavioural change – temper tantrum, being naughty or difficult, tearful or withdrawn. There may only be subtle warnings signs but identification of these signs is essential for every child. This is the key to treating the hypo quickly, and preventing any risk of impairment to the brain.

Case Study

I will never forget the first time my son went hypo. He was six years old, and it happened in the first year of diagnosis after our second routine check-up at the hospital. Instead of buying a sandwich at the hospital I thought we would wait until we got into town. It was a mistake. As I was driving along I looked in my rear-view mirror – Scott seemed to be asleep. I thought this was odd because he had not seemed tired. I woke him up – then when we were about a minute away from the shops I heard this almighty scream from Scott. I looked in my mirror again and this child was jerking, hallucinating and screaming – it was every parent's worst nightmare, something I never want to go through again. He seemed like a child possessed. I rushed into a shop to get him a sugary drink, but he would not take it; his lips remained firmly clenched together. I was shaking like a leaf, but from out of nowhere a woman came along who said she was a diabetic and calmly asked if I had a glucagon injection to give him. I was in such a panic it was the most difficult thing to do to get the injection organized and into him, something none of the books or information sheets ever tell you. We drove off and I flagged down a passing police car who gave us an escort to the hospital. Once we arrived the injection started to take effect and Scott went back to his old self, and in fact asked: 'Dad, what is all the fuss about?'

The first hypo has got to be the worst and unless you are a parent of a child with diabetes it is very hard to understand just what it is like. No other hypo Scott has had has been as bad as the first.

Philip, father of Scott, aged 13

Other studies have revealed that at puberty children begin to respond differently to hypos. The most common signs are:

- hunger
- tiredness
- feeling weak
- feeling warm
- trembling
- palpitations and shaking

Hypos can also vary in severity:

- mild: easily treated with a sugary snack or drink – it may just be that the child's blood glucose level has dipped to just below 3mmol/l
- severe: the child starts to become confused, as well as exhibiting some of the other symptoms above. If this progresses the child lapses into unconsciousness and needs an injection of glucose by a health professional, or glucagon, if available.

Parents should always try and avoid severe hypos; they are potentially damaging to future cognitive ability.

Night-time hypos

It is worth testing your child's blood sugar levels once or twice a month in the middle of the night to see if they are low. Doctors now believe that 7mmol/l is a good target to aim for before bedtime. Research has shown that if blood glucose is low in the morning it is very likely that it has been low in the night, and it is worth the effort to monitor this. Most nocturnal hypos are asymptomatic, and do not wake the child, although in the morning he may be grumpy. Bedwetting is also a clue to night-time hypos. Remember, young children may be in bed for up to 12 hours, and that is a long time without food!

Action to stop a hypo

Your child will soon recover by eating some food which will quickly raise blood sugar levels. A small chocolate bar or a couple of teaspoons of honey will do. Follow up with a carbohydrate-rich snack such as a slice of wholemeal bread, a biscuit or a glass of low-fat milk.

If your child is too confused to eat, rub some fresh fruit jam or honey on his gums. As a last resort an intra-muscular injection of glucagon (which works in the opposite way to insulin) should be given, although be prepared for your child to vomit afterwards. Ask your diabetic team about keeping an emergency syringe on standby. Research among children has shown that if the pre-bed blood test is over 7 mmol/l then a night-time hypo is unlikely. Proteins in a bedtime snack, such as a ham or chicken sandwich, are also thought to lower the risk. Two new snack bars designed to be given just before bed have been launched in America to guard against night-time hypos: NiteBite, marketed by a Massachusetts company, and Zbar, marketed by a firm in Miami. They contain uncooked cornstarch, sucrose and protein and clinical research has found that eating a bar in the evening may reduce night-time and morning hypos by as much as 70 per cent, without increasing the risk of hyperglycaemia.

Another possible precaution is a hypo alarm. These have been available for about 10 years and work by detecting perspiration – one of the symptoms of an adult hypo although there is a question over their reliability. They are currently designed to be worn at night but the only authoritative research has been carried out on adults. However anecdotal evidence suggests that they could be useful for parents worried about their children's ability to identify hypo signs and it may be worth trying one to see how your child responds; it might help to teach him to identify the signs. One of the leading manufacturers is N H Eastwood and Son (*see* 'Useful addresses' at the end of the book).

When treating a hypo, it is worth bearing in mind that low blood sugars can trigger a release of glucose from the liver which makes blood sugars rise again. If you have already given your child a snack to restore blood sugar levels this twin action can cause blood sugar levels to spiral and remain high for some hours. There is then a risk of hyperglycaemia lasting several hours.

Ketoacidosis

This serious condition is a cause of diabetic coma or ketosis, and it signals a relative lack of insulin. It can be triggered by stress, either physical, such as infection, or psychological.

Ketoacidosis is caused by the liver's reaction to extremely low insulin levels in the body, and to the breakdown of fat, resulting in potentially poisonous byproducts called ketones circulating in the blood. Giving insulin and fluids will 'cure' this condition by lowering the blood sugar level and eliminating the toxic ketones.

It is fairly common to find this complication at diagnosis in children. Unless it is swiftly recognized and treated it is a potentially fatal condition.

Long-term complications

A major American study called the Diabetes Control and Complications Trial (DCCT), which was carried out in 29 different centres, has convincingly found that keeping good glycaemic control – that is keeping blood glucose levels as close to normal (non-diabetic) range as possible – can prevent the development of life-threatening complications by as much as 75 per cent. Over a long period of time, poorly controlled and high blood sugar levels can affect the eyesight, circulation, kidneys and feet.

The DCCT's findings are relevant for adolescents but scientists believe that they are difficult to apply to young children mainly because it is extremely rare to find the onset of complications before puberty, and because strict guidelines are too difficult and dangerous to impose upon children. The only danger lies in the cumulative effect on cognitive functioning if a young child has persistent hypos. However, the risk of complications as a result of bad glycaemic control rises sharply once children reach adolescence.

The point that is clear, though, is the importance of maintaining control over your child's blood sugar levels.

In summary

Give yourself some leeway when it comes to monitoring your child's blood sugar levels. Be prepared to take into account illness, fussy eating, temper tantrums, unexpected exercise and their wish to sample their first independence (*see* later chapters). It will make life much more stressful for everyone to be *constantly* worrying about food intake and injections, although it is vital to strive for reasonably good control. If in doubt keep your child's blood sugar levels slightly higher than usual; the main danger with young children is allowing blood sugar levels to fall too low, with the consequence of a hypo. It is useful to keep a supply of glucose tablets or chocolate available for emergencies.

Flexibility is the key to coping with children with diabetes.

Chapter Two

The causes of diabetes

Something happens in one child but not another. It could be a chaotic event, an accumulation of chance things, or simply bad luck having got the right landscape, the landslide starts.

Professor Edwin Gale, London

There are three stages directly linked to the destruction of insulin-making cells in the body, and therefore to the start of diabetes. The first involves the unique, genetic make up of your child. Professor John Todd of the Wellcome Trust Centre for Human Genetics at Oxford University, England, has discovered that diabetes is a genetic disease in as much as almost all cases involve the presence of defective genes. It seems that the more defective genes a child has, the lower the age of onset and the more rapid the destruction of beta-cells. Scientists in Oxford know that there are between 12 and 20 different genes implicated in diabetes. Two different flaws, or mutations in DNA have been identified which indicate a predisposition towards the disease.

The second stage is 'factor X', the unknown trigger, or set of triggers, which initiates or sparks off the disease in a genetically susceptible child, and which causes a slow destruction of the beta-cells. The third is the accelerating agent or the 'final straw'. The current thinking is that an environmental agent could precipitate the disease by attacking, destroying or placing an unmanageable burden on the insulin-making cells in the pancreas.

POSSIBLE TRIGGERS OF DIABETES

Initiators of diabetes

- viral infections
- cow's milk proteins
- nitrates in water or food

Precipitators of diabetes

- frequent infections
- frequent intake of carbohydrates and protein-rich foods
- cold environment
- high growth rate
- stressful life events

▓ VIRUSES

Viruses have been under suspicion as the prime initiators of diabetes for some time.

Current thinking is that the destruction of beta-cells is the result of a number of events, and that a virus or infection could be responsible for either initiating or precipitating the disease. It may be that Type I diabetes is triggered by:

- an initiating virus – an agent which infects a child either in the womb or in the early stages after birth which may be mistakenly identified as 'self' by the body's immature immune system and may therefore remain in the body, slowly attacking pancreatic cells
- a precipitating virus – an infection which triggers diabetes by making such demands on the body's insulin requirements that the already depleted beta-cells are unable to cope, may become the final trigger for the destruction of beta-cells
- a virus directly attacking the beta-cells

■ Which are the risky viruses?

There are a number of viruses which have been linked to the development of diabetes. Prime suspects include the five sub-types of the **Coxsackie b virus**, which cause cold-like symptoms with the added complication of a stomach upset. The difficulty is in identifying this virus, particularly in small babies and children who often seem to lurch from one cold to the next. The Coxsackie viruses bear a remarkable molecular similarity to pancreatic beta-cells, which may provoke the immune system into attacking the insulin-stimulating cells, believing them to be a hostile virus.

Cytomegalovirus has also been associated with diabetes at onset.

Mumps could be a cause. When Finland introduced the MMR vaccination (mumps, measles and rubella) in 1982, mumps was virtually eradicated. Preliminary trials suggested that this may have helped slow down the rate of Type I diabetes, although further studies are underway to study this effect more closely.

Rubella is the cause of diabetes in 10–20 per cent of all children affected by the disease in the womb.

A study in Allegheny County, in the United States, revealed a connection between outbreaks of **chicken pox** and a higher than usual number of reported cases of diabetes two years later. This was backed up by a reported outbreak of diabetes following a chicken pox epidemic in the US Virgin Islands and reports of transient diabetes following chicken pox epidemics in India.

■ COW'S MILK

Proteins in cow's milk are able to cross the immature lining of a baby's gut and filter into the bloodstream, where they are seen as foreign bodies by the developing immune system. Some fractions of milk protein bear a remarkable molecular similarity to beta-cells and the theory is that the baby's undeveloped immune system might mistake the healthy pancreatic cells for milk proteins and attack them as foreign bodies, resulting in their destruction.

But there are other elements to this story. Researchers are looking closely at what happens when a mother gives up breast feeding in favour of formula milk and whether this might be enough to trigger a reaction in some children.

Other factors lending weight to the cow's milk theory are:

- Insulin-dependent diabetes is up to 50 per cent higher among children who are bottle-fed.
- Finland leads the world both in the consumption of milk and in the incidence of diabetes.
- Norwegian and Swedish researchers found that nine years after breast-feeding dropped to an all time low amongst new mothers, the incidence of Type I diabetes rose to an all-time high.
- Breast-feeding reduces the risk of diabetes by two or three times, according to American research. This is because breast-feeding encourages an improved and strengthened immune system in an infant.
- A greater proportion of children with diabetes have received extra cow's milk by the age of three months compared with children who do not have diabetes.

The problem with this theory is that there are many children with Type I diabetes who have been exclusively breast-fed and who have never consumed cow's milk, yet still go on to develop the condition.

NITRATES IN WATER AND FOOD

Nitrates are naturally occurring chemicals and there has been considerable concern in the UK and in the USA over high levels of nitrates in drinking water, a result of the residue of fertilizers used on farmland filtering through rivers into drinking water.

Research has proved that nitrates can alter in the stomach and turn into nitrosamines, compounds which have been shown to induce diabetes in animals by damaging pancreatic beta-cells.

Nitrates enter our systems through contaminated drinking water, vegetables which have absorbed excess nitrates (particularly leafy green vegetables), and preserved fish and meat. Scandinavian countries, which have the highest rates of insulin-dependent diabetes in the world, are also major consumers of smoked fish and mutton. Researchers in Colorado, in the United States, have suggested that there might be a connection between Type I diabetes and consumption of nitrosamine-rich smoked mutton by their parents at the time of conception.

In the United Kingdom researchers in Yorkshire have found a link between high nitrate levels and the development of diabetes in certain areas, and are planning to take this study further.

▨ COLD WEATHER

Studies from around the world have shown that the highest rates of diabetes occur in the coldest months of the year. Cold weather may make extra demands on insulin production in the body and be a 'final straw' in a susceptible child who might have already been affected by a virus. Non-diabetic children have higher blood sugar levels in the winter.

Generally rates of Type I diabetes drop in countries nearer the equator (Asian countries have among the lowest rates in the world). This north–south divide is mirrored in the United Kingdom. The highest number of cases of Type I diabetes are found in Scotland and in Northern Ireland. However there are confusing exceptions – the sun-drenched Mediterranean island of Sardinia, with a population of 1.6 million people, has the second highest rate of Type I diabetes in Europe after Finland, with 30 cases among every 100,000 under the age of 14. And Iceland has far lower rates than its high-level neighbours.

▉ LOW ZINC LEVELS

Zinc levels in the hair, nails and blood are generally found to be lower in children with diabetes than in non-diabetic children. Scientists already know that some metals are present during certain metabolic events in major cells in the body and research has indicated that there may be a link up between low zinc exposure and repeated viral infections.

▉ GENETICS

Certain countries have far higher rates of diabetes than others. For example, Finland, with a population of around 5 million, has the highest rate of insulin-dependent diabetes in the world, averaging 35 cases per 100,000 head of population, and with more boys affected than girls. Asia, Australia, New Zealand and Africa have some of the lowest rates, with less than two affected children in every 100,000 under the age of 20. Recent studies revealed that a child in Finland is 400 times more likely to contract diabetes than one in China, which may demonstrate the different genetic susceptibilities between populations.

Many countries with high numbers of children with diabetes are also reporting more cases in younger children, and it seems certain that something important happens very early in life – probably even in utero – which increases the risk.

▉ OTHER BIRTH FACTORS

A study of 220 mothers with children diagnosed with Type I diabetes in Yorkshire in the UK has found several significant risk factors. Compared with a control group of 400 mothers of healthy children, the survey found that more mothers with diabetic children:

- had had caesarean births
- were over 35
- had experienced pre-eclampsia

The epidemiological group is planning a larger survey to assess if there are certain risk factors in pregnancy and childbirth. Dr Trish McKinney, in charge of the study, says that it was important to find out about environmental factors, as she believes Type I diabetes may be caused by the cumulative effect of a number of triggers in genetically susceptible children.

Diabetes in the family
Mothers suffering from gestational diabetes do not carry any higher risk of passing on diabetes to their child than other mothers, although their babies may be large and at risk of hypoglycaemia or very low blood sugar levels for a short time after delivery.

Genetics do play a part, but only a unique combination from mother and father can cause a child to become susceptible – there would then have to be a further trigger before diabetes developed.

Only 10 per cent of children with diabetes have a diabetic parent, and in these cases diabetes is most commonly passed through the father's genes. There is a 6 per cent risk of contracting diabetes by the age of 20 if your father has Type I diabetes.

CHILD GROWTH AND PUBERTY

Although not directly a cause of diabetes puberty might be one of the accelerating factors. It is known there are certain peak times of diagnosis during childhood which link up with growth spurts. Around 50 per cent of cases are diagnosed before the age of 15, with the main onset period at puberty or around the age of 12. This is the peak time for rapid growth and development, which is associated with increased insulin sensitivity due to high levels of growth hormones circulating at this age. All this rapid growing during the teen years adds heavily to the work of the beta-cells and may therefore accelerate their destruction.

STRESS

Psychological stress has been associated with the onset of Type I diabetes for many years. Stress increases our insulin requirement, and this extra demand could precipitate the onset of diabetes. Research has shown that in many cases a stressful life event occurred a year or so before diagnosis of diabetes in groups of children aged five to nine.

Research in Sweden, published in 1995, suggested that stress as early as before the age of two – even something as common as the effect of parents separating – can have an impact, and increase the risk of Type I diabetes. Stress can be felt by children when there are difficult family relationships or external problems as routine as a change in the family's lifestyle or a move to another part of the country.

Other anecdotal evidence reinforces the view that stress has a part to play. After the 1994 Los Angeles earthquake there was an upsurge in reported cases of diabetes among children in the area. And between 1980 and 1992 the incidence of diabetes in children under the age of 14 in Kuwait shot up by 385 per cent – it was during this time that Iraq invaded the country. Kuwait now has one of the highest incidences of diabetes in the Middle East.

Chapter Three

Helping your child

Case Study
One thing perhaps most of us discover fairly early after diagnosis, whether child, teenager or adult, is that the outside world, the real world, does not make allowances for someone with diabetes.

Jenny, mother of Bev, diagnosed at 5, now 27

Diabetes is a chronic illness which demands huge changes within the family. Few other conditions place such relentlessly high demands on relations between parents and children or require such a high level of medical responsibility from the immediate family .

Health professionals working closely with families now recognize that the emotional impact of coping with diabetes, and the way that is handled, is a fundamental factor in the control of the disease. If there are good coping skills then your child will learn to adapt and live well with the disease. Parents who succeed in managing diabetes work well together, support each other and their child, and search out extra help from health-care teams and from other affected families. This involves parents taking centre stage from the start, and later offering supporting parts to brothers, sisters, grandparents, aunts and uncles before finally allowing the child to go it alone. It also means never being afraid to ask for help. Any family members who come into direct contact with your child should be encouraged to learn as much as possible about diabetes and its physical and psychological impact upon your lives.

Having a child with diabetes presents different kinds of stress at each stage of the child's development, and how you cope can depend on your own physical and psychological strengths. It is not as simple as accepting the condition and getting on with life; you might sail through toddlerhood and reach a crisis when your child becomes an adolescent – or vice versa!

At times of stress there are steps which you can take to help alleviate anxiety and tension, and these are discussed later. Taking care of yourself is just as important as taking care of your children – how you feel will rub off on children. Learning to lighten the burden of diabetes may seem impossible in the early stages after diagnosis, but as you begin to adapt things will improve.

Parents and diabetes
Research has shown that metabolic control in a child with diabetes is good:

- when the child comes from a stable family, with little conflict and stress
- when there is little conflict between parents and child
- when mothers are not overwhelmed with anxiety by the the day-to-day management of their child's diabetes
- when parents co-operate with each other over the management of the diabetes regime

From *Use of a Family Record in Diabetes Clinics* by Dr Jeannette Josse, psychotherapist and family therapist

THE PSYCHOLOGICAL CHALLENGES FACING PARENTS

When diabetes is diagnosed it is quite normal to experience all the symptoms of shock and bereavement: worry, anxiety, depression, sadness and self-blame. Not only are you having to deal with emotional confusion, but you are also having to learn a whole lot of new medical jargon and techniques to ensure that your child remains well.

At the same time as coming to terms with a life-long chronic condition you will have to accept a burden of responsibility beyond any of your previous expectations. You will be confronted with the task of regulating your child's blood sugar levels, giving injections of insulin and supervising (often initially painful) blood tests as well as monitoring food and physical activity every single day – without any let-up.

The confusion you are bound to experience stems from the sudden 'loss' of your child's previously healthy life and all the changes in family routine that you will have to make. This is a quite normal reaction. You are bound to wish it had not happened to your child and worry about the future, especially when people talk about the possible future complications of the disease. If you or your partner already have diabetes then you may experience overwhelming feelings of guilt. Again this is normal; you are feeling vulnerable and trying to find answers.

As a parent you may later fall into the trap of pushing your child in a way which is rather more than simple encouragement. Or you may feel like overcompensating by buying expensive presents to prove that she can actually do many things despite the condition to somehow 'apologize' for the disease. Finding a balance – without being too protective or too pushy – is hard to achieve but is is important for both your child and you.

Diabetes means learning to live with:

- a feeling that you have lost your 'healthy' child
- changes in your family life
- the ever-present threat of future complications
- the task of achieving a balanced life taking into account all the restriction diabetes may impose
- losing a degree of spontaneity in family life

Key questions
Three key questions may loom large in the early days of diagnosis:

- **Can I ensure that my child survives?** Everything will be done to help you in the early stages of diagnosis. The hospital team looking after your child will be there to provide support and information, and diabetic nurse specialists are both an important mine of information and a huge support to families.
- **Will my child be able to live a fulfilling life?** The answer is yes. Insulin injections are a life-saving treatment and mean your child will grow up into a healthy adult with normal expectations. In addition, there is a great deal you can do for your child to boost their health and happiness.
- **How will my child cope?** Children are remarkably resilient and adaptable, and can confidently talk about their diabetes and food requirements, and recognize hypo symptoms from as early as four or five. However they are also sensitive to your anxieties, which can be transferred to them, causing them distress. Counselling or talks with a psychologist trained in diabetes care might help to confront frightening feelings and prepare the ground for a change in behaviour or a more positive approach.

It is normal, and healthy to be upset when your child is diagnosed as having diabetes. But it is not always easy to share those feelings, according to Dr Jeannette Josse, a psychotherapist in Cambridge, England, who was herself diagnosed as having diabetes herself at the age of 18.

She points out that this often becomes harder when parents are praised for 'doing so well' at the clinics. Parents should try to unburden themselves, she believes, and to ask for help by finding people they can talk to about their worries – such as fear of hypos, fear of their child dying, and even fear of injecting their child. There is no shame in feeling vulnerable and asking for help to change either feelings, or certain aspects of behaviour. As with most aspects of diabetes there has to be a balance between asking for help from others and soldiering on regardless of increasing, and mounting, stress.

Positive thinking

Start by believing that diabetes will not prevent you or your child from living a full and active life. Almost all parents who face a diagnosis of diabetes in their child will want to find out as much information about the disease as possible – and make contact with other parents. Specialist nurses are excellent sources of information about parent network groups, or they can simply help by putting one family in touch with another. It can be very reassuring to know that other people have similar feelings and struggles to yourself. Try the British Diabetic Association or the Juvenile Diabetes Federation, with offices in London and New York (*see* 'Useful addresses' at the end of the book). The more you understand about diabetes the more you can help your child so that you both come to terms with the illness.

Parents need to manage diabetes with their own children until they are old enough to manage on their own. It is tempting to take over all your child's tasks because of the diabetes but it will not help her learn to be independent and may even stunt her self-esteem.

In the beginning
There are recognized stages of grief, or of coming to terms with the diagnosis of chronic illness in your child. Each stage might be more or less acute for particular individuals but often the pattern is as follows:

- **shock**, a sense of disbelief, numbness and fear, or an inability to accept what is being said, a reaction which might also be expressed in real physical symptoms
- **anger**, which may be directed towards yourself as a parent through self-blame, or frequent self-questioning, towards the medical team which has made the diagnosis and tells you that there is no cure for this potentially life-threatening condition, or even towards the child because of the tremendous changes a diagnosis of diabetes will make to the whole family
- **sadness**, which may be a symptom of depression which some

parents will continue to experience at different stages of their child's development
- **denial**, a feeling that this really cannot be happening to your family – parents who experience these feelings may, in the early stages, find it hard to follow the insulin regimes
- **guilt**, another common reaction which can in fact help parents mobilize efforts to care for their child, and which will eventually pass
- finally **acceptance**, an ability to adapt to the new circumstances, when the whole family realize that they must get on and co-operate with their new lifelong companion – diabetes

Coping

Coping with diabetes is an ongoing, evolving process for both parent and child. The diagnosis of the condition is the time of greatest upheaval and it is at this stage that the health-care team looking after your child should give you the greatest support. Not only do you have to support and help your child, but you must recognize that you, as a parent, could do with some help .

It is impossible to put a time-scale on full acceptance of diabetes, or indicate when a family will be ready to fully adapt to the changed circumstances, but psychologists suggest that within a year of diagnosis most families will have settled down – although parents who suffer most stress and anxiety in the beginning are likely to need support for longer. Expect new problems to present themselves at each new milestone in your child's development; they all need to be addressed and dealt with. There will be ups and downs as fresh challenges arise, such as illness or the days when your child will not eat.

To summarize:

- Learn as much as possible about the disease and educate your child to her level as you go along.
- Make contact with other families with similarly aged children so that you can discuss different phases and their inherent problems.

- Use the resources of your health-care team and talk about your problems.
- Share the strain – involve all members of the family including grandparents. Do not hide the condition, as the more people who know the easier life will become for both you and your child in terms of acceptance.
- Support your child. Research has found that diabetic children with families who are supportive and stick together manage to control their condition better.

Any parents of a chronically ill child will know about friction in the family – and about friction in their own relationship.

Case Study
The emotional stress on families, and between couples, can be enormous. Doctors and nurses need to understand this so that they can empower parents who do the caring 24 hours a day 52 weeks of the year.

The stress between a couple may be the friction of one parent doing more than the other. One may go out to work and return home and then try to take control, or there may be a power struggle between couples over who is better than the other at caring for the child.

Fathers might go off into denial and there may be blame between the couple. The friction might be heightened by the child manipulating the situation, neglecting to have an injection, refusing to eat.

Sibling rivalry can also be fantastic! I have two boys who have diabetes and one girl in the middle who does not. There have been times when both boys are having a hypo – this middle child can feel ignored, and that her own needs are not being met.

It might help couples to find someone, a third party, to talk to without their partner so that they can open up and express their feelings without the other one being there – it might free them from the inhibition of saying something 'bad' or 'wrong' or disloyal about their partner.

The sad truth is that many couples do split up – and the cause is the stress of having diabetes in the family.

Veronica, mother of Benjamin, aged 16, and Leo, aged 13

THE PSYCHOLOGICAL CHALLENGES FACING CHILDREN

The effect of the diagnosis of diabetes on a child will depend on the child's age and maturity. On a positive note, she will probably have felt ill for some time and will be happy that this is being recognized and dealt with. Insulin therapy will improve matters in the beginning, but it is the long-term acceptance and attitude that will need support and help.

Very young children will find it difficult to understand the changes in their lives, such as painful blood testing and injections. They might think they are being punished or feel ashamed and guilty. Young children will not understand what 'long-term complications' means, and may believe that their parents have the power to take the diabetes away. Or they may use diabetes to exert their control – use hypos as an excuse for bad behaviour or as a means of avoiding something unpleasant.

If a child is disturbed and distressed, this is bound to affect blood glucose levels, which will then heighten stress and tension at home. Diabetic children have to fight a hidden battle – there is nothing external to show that they have diabetes and, as they get older, they have to learn and understand the long-term consequences. They may go through a stage of denying that they have diabetes. This will be hard to accept, but it may be a cry for help from within, a plea for recognition as a complete person rather than being labelled as a 'child with diabetes'. They may also use denial to exert their own personality, to become who they were before diabetes was diagnosed.

Your child will hear about other children doing adventurous, challenging sports or feats, but might well be happy meeting the challenge of leading a normal life. And this, as one parent succinctly put it, is 'as great an achievement for a child or teenager with diabetes as climbing a mountain'.

Some children may also become fearful about what might happen to them in the future, and these fears need to be addressed before they become all-consuming. A child may have heard about a great uncle who died after having his leg amputated because of diabetes; a fear that the same thing may happen to the child can cause the severest anxiety and she will need reassurance. Children with diabetes still face all the same challenges and development stages as healthy children, but having diabetes can be an added negative or positive at each phase. Learning to turn life's challenges into positives is the extra hurdle facing parents and children with diabetes. Children will have to learn how to handle being different, know more about food and exercise than the average child (and their impact upon the body), know about illness from an early stage, and accept that they are not quite like all their friends.

As they grow older they are bound to worry more particularly at adolescence because they discover that having diabetes can be life-threatening. They may feel resentful, and want to test the boundaries by rejecting their condition. They will not want to be seen as different from their peers, and will still want to experiment with drugs, alcohol, smoking and partying all night, just like their friends. They may feel even more pressure than other teenagers to try all these things, to push their bodies to the limit or to take it out on themselves physically. For each child who adapts quickly to a diagnosis of diabetes, there will be another who gets bogged down in a sea of confusion, which might emerge as behavioural or emotional problems such as depression, irritability or withdrawal. Children will also pick up on the way *you* feel from an early stage by watching and sensing your reactions. The way you, as parents, handle the disease from the early days will have a major impact on whether your child eventually manages it in a mature and responsible way.

The question is sometimes raised, whether there is such a

thing as a diabetic personality. The answer is probably not, although some psychologists in the past have suggested such a thing. However what seems certain is that some children do cope better with their diabetes than others, perhaps because of the atmosphere at home or at school, relationships with siblings and parents and their age at diagnosis.

▮ BROTHERS AND SISTERS

All sorts of mixed feelings may emerge among your other, healthy, children when a child is diagnosed with diabetes. The feelings might range from jealousy to worry and fear of 'catching' the same disease. There may be anger, sadness and a feeling of guilt they they are not also affected.

Brothers and sisters who have been questioned about the condition say that they feel left out, alone and ignored and want to be 'centre stage' with their parents. Suddenly the spotlight is on the diabetic child, and the parents might have to be away from the family in hospital. The other children may not fully understand what is going on.

Jealousy can evolve into sibling rivalry and it is best to be aware of this and as things settle down, and new patterns and routines are established, try not to make diabetes a constant focus of difference between the children. For example try making healthy changes to the whole family's diet rather than concentrating solely on what your child with diabetes is eating.

It is important that the whole family knows about the condition, that it is explained, even to the youngest members of the family, in simple, clear language, and that their help is asked for so that they become, and feel, involved. Every member of the family is going to have to learn to adapt to this new diagnosis.

Action

- Ensure that brothers and sisters know as much as they can about diabetes, and reassure them that they will not catch it.
- Answer all questions as truthfully as possible.
- Involve brothers and sisters in any hospital visits.
- Find a job for an interested brother or sister to do – for example to put on a 'show' if some distraction is needed for a blood test or injection.
- Share your feelings with your other children and encourage them to do the same.
- Encourage all members of the family to take blood tests as a show of support.

GRANDPARENTS

Grandparents may go through the same feelings of sadness, disbelief and blame as parents, but they might not to be willing to express them. Most grandparents think their grandchildren are marvellous in every way. They enjoy them in a special way, with more freedom to indulge and less front-line responsibility. So it can be traumatic for a healthy grandparent to find that a very new grandchild has a condition which is lifelong and potentially life-threatening.

Do not forget that grandparents might not know much about diabetes and will need educating too; explain diet restrictions and blood testing even if they only see their grandchildren occasionally. They will also have to learn the art of treating your child with diabetes in the same way as they treat their other grandchildren. Other children may feel ignored and resentful if the child with diabetes is favoured.

Grandparents and diabetes
Winthrop University Hospital in the United States held an educational programme for grandparents of children under the age of six who had diabetes. They learned about injections, food,

hypos and glucagon. None of the grandparents in the survey had ever provided overnight care but 50 per cent had looked after the grandchild during the day. After three months none had 'graduated' to night-time care. Two main reasons were given: distance from the child's home and the parents' fear of allowing others to care for their child over night.

However the conclusion was that most grandparents felt much more confident and able to look after their grandchild, especially if an emergency arose, and they all felt the benefit of talking to other grandparents.

DIVORCED PARENTS

If you are separated from the mother or father of your child but still maintain contact, it is important to work out a plan of action so that diabetes is not used as a point of conflict. If your child receives extra treats at your ex-partner's home at the weekends it will do nothing to help control the condition, and it compounds the problem if there are rows about it in front of your child.

There will inevitably be different rules at different homes, but your child needs to feel safe and cared for, and one set of guidelines for the management of diabetes is the ideal solution to this problem.

Action

- Keep a bag with all the diabetes paraphernalia so that it is taken to both parents' homes rather than having a set in each.
- Make sure the 'house rules' for food, meal times and injection routines are kept the same as far as possible.
- Communicate with each other, even if the subject is solely your child's diabetes.
- Try and avoid conflicts or rows about diabetes care in front of your child. This can instil feelings of guilt or a sense that your child is somehow responsible for the divorce or separation or even the diabetes.

- Make sure you are both competent at handling injections, and know exactly who to contact and where in the event of an emergency or a severe hypo.

COUNSELLING

Counselling is a means of helping you to help yourself by exploring problems and encouraging you to make decisions about what to do next. But counsellors will not make decisions for you, so do not expect them to provide their own solutions to any conflicts – that will have to come from you.

Counsellors have the skills to listen, empathize with your problems and enable you to understand more about them. Family counselling is useful for those who cannot offer each other the support they need and require help in tackling specific relationship problems.

Families experiencing stress and difficulty or finding it hard to cope with a particular stage of their child's development, may find counselling or family therapy helpful. A talk with a therapist might also be useful if a family is locked into a pattern of negative behaviour. A therapist can pinpoint areas of stress and strain and then teach the skills to help alter these patterns. Your family may benefit from counselling or family therapy sessions if:

- there are constant conflicts and rows
- tantrums, anger and tears break out regularly over small issues
- behavioural problems emerge, even minor ones such as your child refusing to stay overnight with a friend because of a fear of what will happen to her diabetes control
- your child becomes withdrawn
- any member of the family feels acute anxiety about diabetes

Not every family with a child with diabetes needs counselling, however, and in some cases it can be the wrong approach, unnecessarily heightening the anxiety about the condition within the family.

Family therapists

These specialist therapists are experts on family relationships, and offer the whole family the opportunity to talk through their feelings of stress and anxiety with a third party. They usually see the whole family together and can help resolve conflicts. The counsellor may offer ways of coping, and of changing patterns of behaviour, although the final resolution of underlying problems will remain with you. Talking through the way you feel is very therapeutic, and can alleviate many of the pressurized feelings associated with stress.

Psychotherapists

Psychotherapists can offer ways of changing patterns of behaviour. For example they may help a child overcome needle phobia, which can develop because of a cycle of anxiety and tension which builds up before injection time. This cycle may start at breakfast when a child is reminded that it is injection time. It might be made worse if everyone is in a hurry in the morning to get to work, school, college. Tensions slowly rise with ever more reminders until the moment of injection – and pain. In an extreme case the child might cry helplessly behind the sofa, refusing to come out and confront the parent, who has probably become very tense and cross and anxious about hypos.

A psychotherapist will suggest new ways of taking the heat out of the situation such as someone else taking over the injections for a while, or distracting the child with TV or a story to reduce any mounting tension. The overall aim will be to defuse the situation, so that the tension is lifted.

A psychotherapist might be able to offer behavioural therapy, a simple course of treatment in which the child's anxieties are confronted. Relaxation techniques are used, and the child will be encouraged to look at pictures or hold a needle (under supervision) to allay any fears in a very relaxed way.

One of the biggest problem areas is blood glucose testing.

Reacting against blood testing is common but it may simply be a phase, and you might have to accept that for a while blood testing will have to be kept to a minimum. Making demands and getting fraught will not help – it will only make matters far worse. You will have to learn the art of compromise with older children and teenagers. Set aside certain days or times for blood testing, even if, at first, it is as little as twice a week, and aim to build up confidence and allow your child a say in doing these tests.

Conflicts

Diabetes is a hidden condition, and this fact can become a source of conflict. A diabetic child looks no different on the outside from any other child of the same age and this can lead to the following problems:

- You will want your child to be independent, but also seek help for a hypo.
- You will not want your child to feel isolated or alone but she may not want to talk about the diabetes.
- You will be grateful for all the help your diabetes clinic gives you, but might feel resentment that you and your child have to attend.

Remember that having diabetes is not just about injections, diet and insulin – it is about the whole person.

THERAPIES FOR PARENTS

Parents of children with diabetes face particular pressures. They have to become their child's own doctor, to watch for the danger signs of illness or complications. It is an all-consuming responsibility with little let-up. But it is vital for parents to find time for themselves, to look after their mind, body and emotions. In this section therapies suitable for parents of children with diabetes are suggested which, it is hoped, will become small refuges from the day-to-day stresses and strains of caring for a sick child.

The key is to maintain a feeling of balance, and of being in control. But you also need time out to take stock and recharge your inner emotional batteries. Relaxation techniques such as meditation and yoga will help to induce an overall sense of wellbeing and can offer a welcome sanctuary from the daily regimes imposed by diabetes. Do not feel guilty about needing this time out – it will strengthen your resolve to manage the diabetes successfully until your child is old enough to manage alone.

If life suddenly seems full of problems and you are unable to cope you will probably start suffering the first symptoms of stress. Excessive stress leads to anxiety, which can then lead on to depression.

RECOGNIZING STRESS

Short-term effects of stress

- tense muscles
- edginess and 'butterflies'
- need to urinate more often
- sweaty hands
- faster breathing

Long-term effects of stress

- headaches
- leg aches
- heart disease and high blood pressure
- indigestion and ulcers
- poor circulation
- feelings of cold
- skin problems
- insomnia and loss of appetite

Meditation

Meditation can ease stress and anxiety, and help overcome headaches, insomnia and tension. Research has shown that meditation will slow the heartbeat and dissolve feelings of stress and tension. It can induce deep rest and alleviate depression.

If you have never meditated before then it may be best to find a teacher. Otherwise tapes can be useful. Read as much as possible about the subject before you start. The ideal environment is one of peace and tranquillity in which you can clear your mind of all stimulating thoughts. Using a mantra – a word repeated over and over – can encouage this calm internal atmosphere.

Establish a slow rhythm with the chant (one word such as 'one' or 'om') and focus on your breathing. Looking at a candle or picture can help. After a while, and with practice, meditation will bring about an inner calm and sense of deep relaxation.

Yoga

Yoga can specifically help:

- fatigue
- insomnia
- headaches
- the balance of the nervous system
- anxiety
- depression

Yoga is a combination of gentle exercise and techniques which act on your mind and emotions. It will teach you how to manage your stress as well as encouraging a more flexible body.

The study of true yoga incorporates meditation. Simple, gentle postures and breathing exercises relax tense muscles, mobilize joints, massage internal organs and tone the immune system. They can also strengthen your mental balance. Yoga therapy promotes the body's own natural healing. The most widely available form of yoga is hatha yoga, which covers the postures and exercises and should be practised together with relaxation and breathing exercises, whereas yoga therapy targets specific ailments.

Acupuncture

The power of acupuncture in healing and helping to maintain a balance both physically and mentally is now well recognized in the West.

An acupuncturist will select treatment points on the body and insert fine needles to enhance the flow of chi, the life force. Acupuncture can help calm the emotions and open up blocked meridians – energy channels which run under the skin – to relieve feelings of stress and anxiety. Acupuncture is also very helpful for specific ailments, including pain or joint problems.

Acupressure

This is application of pressure on the same points used for acupuncture, but using fingers rather than needles. There are a number of variations, amongst them shiatsu, a Japanese word meaning 'finger pressure'.

Applying pressure to certain points on the body stimulates the circulation and the hormonal system. Many patients report feelings of deep relaxation after sessions of acupressure.

Massage

A regular body massage will encourage a feeling of overall wellbeing and boost your general health as well as relaxing both body and mind, restoring a sense of balance to the world. There are different techniques used by different practitioners: slow, stroking movements, kneading, knuckling and pressuring are just some of the methods which reduce stress and encourage deep mental and physical relaxation.

▓ Other relaxing therapies

There are many different types of relaxation therapy. You may have your own preference – for example a warm scented bath, followed by a cup of soothing herbal tea and an early night! Specific relaxation therapies include:

- **Flotation.** Floating in a totally enclosed tank of salt water creates a wonderful feeling of weightlessness.
- **Biofeedback.** This involves a series of relaxation exercises, after which the response is monitored by a machine which assess heart rate and muscle tension. It teaches understanding and recognition of your own stress signals.
- **Autogenics.** There are six exercises which teach you how to relax and deal with stress build-up in the body.
- **Visualization.** This encourages the use of soothing pictures to restore wellbeing and feelings of deep relaxation.
- **Art, music and drama therapy.** These stimulate an interest outside the self and relax the mind or draw out emotions and recognize conflict. They are also helpful for putting stressful situations into perspective, giving you an opportunity to express your feelings if words are not enough. Art therapy can give form and shape to inner feelings, while dramatherapy can inspire personal growth – a sense of meaning can be gained through symbolic play-acting or the use of stories, images, music and movement.
- **Spiritual healing.** This brings together mind, body and spirit and encourages you to take your intuition and personal spirituality seriously. Help can be given through relaxation and positive thinking, and it encourages you to be responsible for the way you respond to what happens to you.
- **T'ai chi.** This is a system of slow-moving circular exercises which can be designed to help stress relief. It is a non-combative martial art with the added benefit of meditation and exercise to promote total health and wellbeing.
- **Aromatherapy.** This can release built-up feelings of grief, anger and sadness.

Chapter Four

Diet and nutrition

A HEALTHY DIET

Food is the cornerstone of your child's health on a day-to-day basis. The power and influence of food for a child with diabetes is fundamental. Good food and nutrition will improve your child's quality of life, improve response to treatments of both an orthodox and a complementary sort, as well as providing the essential 'building blocks' for future strength, growth and ability to combat disease.

A healthy diet for children with diabetes over the age of five follows the general guidelines of low fat, high carbohydrate and fibre, and low sugar. There are two important aspects to your child's diet:

- helping control blood glucose levels
- promoting growth

A particularly sensible diet to follow is the one advocated by the British Diabetic Association, which suggests that over half of your child's daily diet should consist of good-quality high-fibre carbohydrate, and 30 per cent of energy requirements should be met by fat or monounsaturated oils such as olive oil. This diet suggests replacing white bread with wholemeal, and emphasizes the use of wholemeal pasta, brown rice, lentils and beans as providing the basic foundation of 'good' carbohydrate. By following this diet it may be possible to achieve a small reduction in insulin while still maintaining good metabolic control.

A high-fibre diet

A survey of ten children on a high-fibre diet providing 60g of fibre and a total of 55 per cent energy intake as carbohydrate, 30 per cent as fat and 15 per cent as protein showed an improvement in blood glucose control over just six weeks. The British Diabetic Association says in a report on diet for children and young people that a high-fibre diet might allow a small reduction in insulin while still maintaining good metabolic control.

Good-quality high-fibre foods include:

- wholemeal pasta
- wholemeal bread
- brown rice
- high-fibre bran-enriched cereals
- pulses, lentils and beans
- jacket potatoes
- oatcakes
- whole (with skin) fresh fruit
- vegetables such as corn on the cob and peas

One important aspect of nutrition is to try always to use fresh, organic fruit and vegetables whenever possible. Chemicals are sprayed on food at every stage from seed to supermarket, so find a reputable supplier of organically grown food – or better still, grow your own. The chemicals used on most food may be considered harmless in small quantities, but the accumulation of the toxins from the chemicals in your child's body should be avoided if possible. These agents or substances impose added burdens on a body which already faces a tough time responding to the demands of diabetes.

The best advice is to find and use food in as near a natural, unpolluted condition as possible. Avoid processed, tinned, frozen, pre-cooked or packaged meals. Try and encourage your child to eat raw foods whenever possible and add sprouting beans and other pulses and grains to the diet.

Carbohydrate is taken into the body as sugar or sucrose and as unrefined carbohydrate from foods such as wholemeal bread, bran cereals, wholemeal or granary biscuits, rye crackers, fruit such as bananas, grapes, pineapple and dried fruits, vegetables like beans and potatoes and bioyoghurts. Over-indulgence in refined sugar should never be encouraged, but it is safe to include a small amount and it may sometimes help to make your child's diet more palatable. Use natural sweetening agents where possible, and encourage children to enjoy the natural sweetness in fruits rather than fruit sweets.

So remember:

• Simple sugars found in sweets and chocolate bars increase blood sugar levels within minutes of eating them so it is only logical that an excess of sweets and sugar is disastrous for diabetes control. However, they do not have to be completely ruled out.
• Starchy carbohydrates such as wholemeal bread, pasta and jacket potatoes also raise blood glucose levels but over several hours. Fibre has the added benefit of slowing the absorption of glucose from the stomach into the blood.
• One gram of fat can release twice as much energy as 1g of carbohydrate or protein, which is why fat should be reduced to around 30 per cent of total energy intake for children.

A family shopping guide and eating routines

• low-fat spreads
• low-fat snacks such as bread sticks, pretzels or non-coated popcorn
• cold-pressed extra virgin olive oil rather than butter or margarine (avoid blended vegetable oils)
• brown/wholemeal/bran loaves rather than white bread
• lentils, pulses, and grains such as couscous or brown rice
• tofu as an alternative for quick stir-fries
• novel fresh fruits such as starfruit, kiwis, mangoes and pineapples to make the fruit bowl look more attractive
• low-fat yoghurt

- light fromage frais instead of full-fat cream

Offer vegetarian meals once or twice a week – a good vegetable stir-fry flavoured with soy sauce or chilli, for example.

The timing of meals is important for children with diabetes. Meal should, ideally, be regularly spaced through the day and include a range of wholesome and nutritious food. Friends, relatives, teachers and club or sports instructors should all understand how important regular meals – and in-between snacks – are to your child. Snacks are often high in calories and fat, so choose fresh fruit, wholewheat crispbreads and high-fibre foods such as oatcakes or bran cereal bars which release energy slowly through the day.

Other factors which have to be taken into acount are:

- moods
- activities
- lifestyle

It is hard to confine children to a strict routine of food when they are faced with a busy schedule that involves school, games and/or dancing classes, as well as socializing with friends. A flexible approach is needed to take into account, for example, extra carbohydrate required to 'cover' any extra exercise, or the extra energy requirements of a school test.

Christmas, birthdays and feast days should not be too hard to manage if diabetes is generally well controlled. There are opportunities to use chocolate as a treat before sport, which will help normalize your child's diet, and there should be no problem allowing moderate amounts of ordinary party food on special occasions, especially if your child is likely to be using up a lot of energy with party games.

Extra vitamins and minerals

You might consider providing vitamin C and B supplements, zinc, magnesium, potassium and chromium. Boosting your child's diet with vitamins and minerals which play a part in insulin production will help to strengthen the system.

Chromium is an essential trace mineral for general health and wellbeing; together with insulin it regulates blood sugar levels and helps to make insulin work more efficiently. The amount of chromium found in the diet differs from country to country, but in general northern European diets are severely deficient. The best natural sources of chromium are cereals, peas and beans, nuts and brewer's yeast, wholemeal products and shellfish (especially mussels).

The way food is prepared can affect its chromium content. Heating results in a significant loss and frozen foods contain little or no chromium. A diet rich in fibre improves the body's ability to absorb and use chromium.

Zinc is another essential trace mineral which helps to facilitate metabolic processes and is needed to assist the release of insulin from any remaining beta-cells in the pancreas. Natural sources are liver, fish and eggs.

Selenium is a vital mineral which works together with vitamins A, B, C and E to defend and improve the body's immune system.

If an older child has poor glycaemic control, try supplementing the diet with **magnesium** for a trial period. A lack of magnesium in the diet has been shown to play a role in insulin resistance; it is a vital mineral for the performance of all cells, and is generally stored in the muscles and bone mass.

▩ EXERCISE AND FOOD

Exercise complements a healthy, well-balanced lifestyle and will also encourage

- an improved attitude to diabetes
- a reduction in the amount of insulin required

However any diet and exercise programme will have to be

carefully monitored, especially in the early days, as it will be important to balance food intake with exercise.

The first thing is to choose a form of exercise that your child really enjoys. The most important point to remember is that there really are no limits – anything from swimming to hockey, from squash to roller-blading has the potential to improve children's co-ordination, boost their self esteem, keep a healthy weight balance and provide them with an all-important feeling of health and wellbeing. Enjoying sport with other children will also stop them feeling different.

Choose anything which exercises the heart, lungs and circulatory system. Among the forms of exercise children with diabetes might enjoy are:

- walking
- running
- swimming
- cycling

Girls are more likely than boys to give up intense exercise in their teens and then begin to worry about putting on weight, so advice on diet and eating habits is a vital part of a keep-fit programme.

Striking the right balance between insulin, exercise and food can be a real challenge, and it may involve blood testing before the start of any exercise, during the activity and afterwards, to monitor how the body copes. Children who are diagnosed in early childhood will probably be aware of how vital it is to check blood glucose levels before and after sport. This applies even more during the teen years, when blood sugar levels may be fluctuating for other reasons.

To summarize:

- Eat a snack before exercise begins.
- Test blood sugar levels at the start.
- Eat a meal of starchy wholesome carbohydrate if the workout has been strenuous.

The effect of exercise can last over a day or two, so if a new sports regime is started, it is worth doing extra blood tests over the following 48 hours.

Case Study

Jane Dillon-Kitz is now grown up. She is a computer sales representative in Connecticut, USA, and has a busy working life, but she became insulin dependent at the age of eight.

As a teenager Jane recalls a constant battle with both her weight and her blood glucose levels. It literally all changed when she took up exercise, she says. She has been working out every day since her teens – weight-training, playing tennis, jogging or using a step machine – and since she took up regular exercise her blood sugar has levelled out and become much more manageable. 'I don't know how people live without exercise. It is a very important part of my life now,' she says.

Courtesy of JDF Countdown Magazine

One of the side-effects of exercising is a surge in blood sugar levels following workouts. During exercise the body draws glycogen from the muscles to fuel muscle movement; at the same time a burst of adrenalin from the adrenal glands prompts the liver to release more glucose. This burst of glucose can fool you into believing that your child needs extra insulin; but this is not necessarily the right course of action. After the initial 'high' there will be a drop in blood sugar levels that can last 24 hours or more. So if extra insulin is taken immediately after exercising then your child might be at risk of a hypo.

It is a matter of trial and error in the beginning. Some older children and teenagers find that after intense exercise, and once their 'high' has levelled out, there is a drop in glucose levels that can last right through the next day. When this is recognized, it can be very helpful in keeping blood sugars low and controlling them.

Exercise will affect your child in a very individual way, but if exercise is a regular feature of his weekly schedule then a pattern will emerge, and you will soon begin to see a clear picture of the body's response.

Finally, here are a few more guidelines:

- Try to encourage your child to take some form of exercise an hour after a meal, when blood sugar levels are at their highest.
- Give your child a small snack such as a drink of fruit juice before exercising and take a carbohydrate 'pick-me-up' along as well, just in case.
- Do not inject insulin into the part of the body that will be exercising. It will be absorbed much faster than usual.

Diet and exercise

Gill Regan, a former Commonwealth Games long jumper and now a professional dietitian on the Nutrition Steering Group of the British Olympic Association, is also Chief Paediatric Dietitian for the Glanhafren NHS Trust in South Wales. She has made a study of the relationship between food, sport and children with diabetes, and she has come up with an eating programme for them along the same lines as a nutrition programme she has devised for top athletes competing at the Olympics.

She has conducted a survey to find out which foods help to maintain blood sugar at a good level two hours after exercise, and are therefore the best hypo preventatives. During the trial she also found that the way the children used available energy depended on their fitness – those who were the fittest appeared to have the best blood sugar levels, while those who had to work hard during exercise sessions used up more energy.

Gill suggests that children benefit from 20g of carbohydrate for every 30 minutes of exercise they do. The carbohydrate programme she devises for athletes is based on the balance between energy required and carbohydrate intake – just as it is in the diet of a child with diabetes.

'Telling the children they have the same diet as an Olympic athlete really helps to sell them the idea,' she says.

Chapter Five

Orthodox treatments

It is important to understand the treatments that your doctor will provide for your child. Not only will you and your child be required to play an active part in any of the treatments, but knowledge will also empower you and enable you to feel in control – one of the most important things for you.

The diagnosis of Type I diabetes will be confirmed by either your doctor, or a hospital diabetic team. Blood and urine tests are usually enough to confirm the diagnosis. Once a diagnosis is made your child is entitled to see a specialist trained in diabetes; every area should have at least one specialist paediatrician skilled in diabetes care.

There are a number of people who will become involved in your child's care.

They are:

- a paediatrician/child specialist
- a dietitian/nutritionist
- a doctor specializing in diabetes/diabetologist
- a chiropodist/foot specialist
- a diabetes nurse specialist
- your own doctor/medical practitioner

Once Type I diabetes is diagnosed the only way forward is a prescription of insulin – for life. However, you can do a lot for your child by introducing complementary therapies from an early stage to work in tandem with the orthodox treatment. Children respond especially well to complementary therapies because their bodies are untainted by years of pollution.

Although every emphasis is placed on good glucose control, you can only do your best, and flexibility is needed both in practical ways and in understanding that sometimes your child will be difficult and unco-operative. At these times try a soothing therapy, such as aromatherapy, which will have a calming influence at a time of stress.

Accept that glucose control can never be perfect but be reassured that injecting will be good enough to maintain your child's health until you all settle down into a routine.

INSULIN

Insulin . . . the very precise and beautiful treatment by which we have been restored to normality . . .

H G Wells, in a letter to *The Times*, 1934

When insulin is injected into the body to replace the lost supply, insulin function is restored. Insulin is not technically a medicine, but a hormone which controls the body's use of food. Its use is not a cure, but a life-saving treatment, which enables your child to stay alive and metabolize food correctly. Without insulin your child would eventually suffer serious weight loss and dehydration, and eventually slip into a coma. If blood sugar levels are allowed to fluctuate wildly with little or no control once your child has reached puberty, there is a risk of future complications affecting major organs, nerves, eyes and feet. Most worryingly, rampant and prolonged poor control may affect the developing intellect and growth in younger children. *If insulin is stopped or the dosage altered without advice from a doctor, your child's immediate and future health could be affected.*

There are at least 300 types of insulin, each with different characteristics, available around the world. Basically they work for different periods of time, and in simple terms they can be broken down into:

- **short-acting** or 'clear' insulins which start to work between 10–30 minutes after injecting and whose effect (one of reducing glucose levels in the blood) lasts for up to eight hours – they can be used alone, when insulin needs are changing, or mixed with other longer-lasting types
- **medium-acting** or 'cloudy' insulins, which work between 25 minutes and one hour after injecting, but whose effect lasts for up to 20 hours
- **long-acting**, also cloudy, insulin, which starts working two to four hours after injecting and lasts up to 28 hours
- a new **fast-acting** insulin which has recently been awarded a drugs licence may be injected immediately before or during a meal, peaks about 60 minutes after injection and lasts about 5–6 hours.

Short-acting insulin 'peaks' between one and four hours after use, and the aim is to give 'cover' for meals taken during that time. Short-acting insulin is designed to be injected 20–30 minutes before food, to give cover solely for that meal.

Paediatricians usually start a newly diagnosed child on a prescription mix of short- and medium-acting insulin, with injections twice a day. This provides immediate cover and a degree of 'follow-on' cover for the rest of the day or night. Insulin doses are measured in units. The more units given the greater the effect on lowering blood sugar levels. Small children may start on only one or two units.

There are a number of factors which will influence how well your child responds to insulin:

- diet and exercise
- lifestyle
- emotions and stress
- age (growth hormones can interfere with insulin action)
- illness
- the use of complementary therapies such as Ayurvedic medicine, traditional Chinese remedies, homeopathy, healing and naturopathy to support the body and promote internal

healing, and relaxing therapies such as yoga, meditation, aromatherapy and reflexology which can also help manage the day-to-day stresses of diabetes and encourage a healthy mental acceptance of the condition

In a child without diabetes, blood glucose levels are carefully regulated by body hormones and remain between 4 and 7 mmol/l. This represents the amount of glucose in the blood and is achieved by balancing the glucose entering the bloodstream as food with that leaving it as energy.

Under normal circumstances the sugar in the blood comes from sugar and carbohydrate in the diet. This is converted into energy and any 'left overs' are stored as glycogen in the liver, or as fat. Insulin is also vital for this conversion. In a healthy child insulin is secreted from the pancreas as a meal is eaten allowing sugar from the meal to penetrate the body cells to give them energy. This goes on for about two hours until insulin and blood sugar levels return to a plateau. Exercise is also part of the equation.

As a general rule:

• food makes glucose levels rise
• insulin and exercise make it fall

A child with diabetes needs an artificial supply of insulin to keep the body healthy to carry out all these different processes. The skill of the specialists is finding a way of delivering insulin which follows, as much as possible, the body's natural cycle and secretions.

In the beginning, take advice from your medical practitioner over which is the best type of insulin for your child; you have every right to request a change later, once things have settled down and you know where you stand. It may be a question of trial and error at first. Insulin will begin to balance your child's blood sugar levels and eliminate the distressing symptoms of the disease, but you may need to 'fine tune' the dose or the type later on.

As you go along you may find that you have to weigh up the pros and cons of animal versus human insulin or the benefits of long-acting insulin against those of medium- or longer-acting insulins which can be given just before meals. And as you develop a greater understanding of blood sugars, diet and exercise, and how they all interact, and more specifically how your child individually responds to insulin treatment, you will become more confident about exploring the different options.

Insulin
The first person to receive insulin was a 14-year-old Canadian boy named Leonard Thompson, who was given a 7.5ml injection of impure extract of ox pancreas into each buttock in January 1922. This did very little to reduce his blood sugar levels, but fortunately for Leonard and thousands of children since, a purer pancreatic extract was produced within a month!
The work of insulin is to:

- help glucose cross the cell membrane and enter cells
- stimulate the liver's manufacture of glycogen
- stop the excessive breakdown of fats
      (with thanks to Dr Peter Swift, Leicester Royal Infirmary)

HOSPITAL VERSUS HOME CARE

There is a chance that in the first days after diagnosis your child will be admitted to hospital while blood glucose levels are stabilized. Alternatively, your child may be treated at home with paediatric nurses trained in diabetes care visiting regularly over the first few weeks. A study by researchers at the University of Leicester, UK, has confirmed that most newly diagnosed children can be managed safely at home, without admission to hospital, but only if senior doctors or diabetic nurse specialists are available to supervise the first injections. The study also found that children managed at home were subsequently admitted to hospital on fewer occasions, and achieved equally good glucose control compared to those who were initially admitted to hospital. So it is possible to avoid the confusion and stress which sometimes occurs with admission to a large hospital. Managing diabetes at home from the start puts you in control, but there will still be regular contact at a specialist clinic with the diabetes team.

You may be overwhelmed with information during your early consultations at the clinic or hospital, so go prepared with any questions (write them down at home as you think of them). Do not worry if some of the questions sound petty or silly. Your consultant should understand all your worries. And do not be afraid to repeat the question if something is unclear or ask the doctor for a written explanation if possible. It might help to make notes of the answers so that you can go through the information again at home. It may help to attend with a friend, relative or partner – if there are two of you at a consultation it will be easier to remember later what has been said.

In the early months of treatment there may be a short-term recovery. At diagnosis there may well be some insulin-producing cells still active in your child's pancreas and the need for insulin may lessen for a while. This is an ideal time to consult a naturopath, who will look at how nutrition can boost your child's health and strengthen the body's ability to 'hold on to' the last remaining functioning pancreatic cells, encouraging them to work effectively for longer.

INJECTING YOUR CHILD

Most parents are daunted by the prospect of their child's first injection of insulin. This first step physically represents a lifetime of injections and emotionally represents the loss of the 'healthy' child. It is bound to be emotionally charged and nerve-wracking, but do bear in mind that the first injection will be done by a health professional who should make every effort to show you and your child that it is not a traumatic event.

Practical tips on preparing for the first injection

- Make sure you are both in a calm, confident frame of mind.
- Do not be in a hurry.
- Approach from the side, giving your child only a brief chance to see the needle.
- Sit with your arm wrapped around your child, in a cuddling position.
- If you are admitted to hospital with your child try and use the time to learn about the different insulins, and ask to be allowed to mix up a dose.
- Pinch up a soft fold of skin and with the needle at an angle of 90 degrees inject into this site, gently keeping the skin held in this fold as you proceed.
- It is important to rotate injection sites – ask about getting a poster of the body to keep at home. Your child can use stickers to highlight the different injection sites.
- Bear in mind that a UK survey carried out by Dr Peter Swift, a consultant paediatrician, which involved 200 children found that 45 per cent were injecting themselves by the age of seven or eight, and 87 per cent by the age of ten!
- The more calm and confident you are, the more your child will want to take over.

Looking after insulin

Insulin is a protein which cannot be taken by mouth so the only sure way of getting the life-saving hormone into the body is by daily injection. Very fine needles and pen injectors are available for babies and young children, which make the process virtually pain free.

Insulin comes in a powder and once it is mixed in water becomes vulnerable to breakdown – which is accelerated by exposure to light and heat, agitation and shaking – so it is not a good idea to keep a vial too long in a handbag. Vials stored out of the refrigerator should be used within 28 days, but in the refrigerator they can be kept for up to three months.

Although there is no alternative to injections yet, work is underway in the United States and the United Kingdom to develop insulin nasal sprays, skin patches and needleless injectors.

■ Can different insulins affect hypos?

Some campaigning groups believe that laboratory-made insulins known as 'human insulins' can mask the symptoms of a hypo in some people. Organizations such as the UK's Insulin Dependent Diabetes Trust, the Swiss Association and the Canadian Alberta Committee for Diabetic Rights are campaigning for more public awareness over this issue and want to see major pharmaceutical companies make animal insulins (derived from the pancreases of pigs and cows) more readily available.

It is probably true that a small number of people do better on animal rather than human insulins, although the view is only supported by anecdotal case histories collected by organizations such as those mentioned above. But it is quite usual to begin a newly diagnosed child's treatment with human insulin.

■ BLOOD TESTS

In the early days of diagnosis many regular blood tests should be done to check on blood glucose levels and to see whether with the new prescription is working for your child. It can be painful – most children dread the blood test more than the daily injections.

The only tried and trusted method of diagnosing accurate blood glucose levels is by pricking a finger with a needle and placing a drop of blood on a diagnostic strip which is in turn placed into a small, hand-held monitoring device. The concentration of blood glucose is analysed by a colour change on the test strip. In most countries, except the United States, this is now measured in millimoles per litre – written mmol/l. In the

United States the old measure of milligram per decilitre, or mg/dl, is still used.

The WHO guidelines
The World Health Organization guidelines say that diabetes is confirmed when the glucose levels in the blood are over 11 mmol/l during a glucose tolerance test. In some out of control diabetes the levels can soar as high as 30mmol/l. Guidelines from the British Diabetic Association say that the ideal level is between 4 and 7 mmol/l.

THE FUTURE

There are many biotechnology companies hoping to become the first to set the market alight with new methods of blood testing and delivering insulin in a more comfortable, pain-free way. The ultimate goal is a device which includes constant glucose monitoring with the appropriate delivery of insulin as an automatic response – all pain free and easy to manage

Amlyn therapy

Amlyn is another hormone produced in the same beta-cells as insulin, and was discovered in 1987. A San Diego-based company has developed a chemical analogue of human amlyn and maintains that taking it with insulin helps glucose control. Clinical trials are ongoing and if they are successful the company hopes to file an American Food and Drug Administration application in 1998.

Ceramic beads

Researchers in California are currently testing a new method of delivering insulin. Dr Edward Pope from the Matech Company has devised a system of enclosing insulin in tiny pink ceramic beads which may, in the future, be inserted into a patient's stomach or under the skin during a small operation. The walls of the beads are porous, with microscopic holes just large enough to allow glucose molecules from the bloodstream to enter and trigger the cells in the beads into producing insulin. Dr Pope believes it might be possible to deliver a year's supply of insulin this way and his work has received backing from the American government. Trials are expected to begin in 1998.

Orthodox preventative therapies

Blood tests are in place which can usefully predict whether a child is at risk of developing diabetes.

Predictor tests for diabetes
New tests developed in the past decade can give doctors a clear idea of who will go on to develop diabetes – before any symptoms occur. There are three tests:

- The ICA (islet cell auto antibodies) test measures the level of beta-cell antibodies present in the bloodstream.
- The insulin auto antibodies test measures antibodies produced by the body against its own insulin.
- The first-phase insulin release test is an intravenous glucose test which can measure the degree of damage that has already occurred in the pancreas.

Using these three tests doctors can judge the percentage likelihood of a child going on to develop Type I diabetes within the next five years. In the United States the tests are being used in a national screening programme as part of the National Institutes of Health Diabetes Prevention Trial, which encourages relatives aged from 3 to 45 to take a test. Those that test positive may be entered into the trial which is looking at whether insulin given orally or by injection can delay the onset of diabetes in these susceptible people.

These tests are not yet widely offered, but there are trials assessing different possible preventative treatments underway, including the following.

Nicotinamide

A total of 24 European countries, together with Canada and the United States, have joined together to take part in the European Nicotinamide Diabetes Intervention Trial (ENDIT). Nicotinamide is one of the B group of vitamins. Small amounts are found in a healthy diet (in foods such as yeast, lean meat, liver and chicken with lesser amounts in milk and leafy green vegetables), and early tests have shown that high doses may protect beta-cells from attack by the body's immune system. Over 500 relatives of Type I patients are being recruited whose antibody tests are positive – that is they are at risk of developing Type I diabetes. The ENDIT trial uses high doses of highly purified nicotinamide, and the results of the trial are expected by the year 2000.

Insulin therapy

A seven-year trial has been launched in the United States to establish whether treating children with insulin before the onset of diabetes can be a successful therapy. Predictor tests pick up those at risk of developing the disease, and these children and adults are recruited into the study. There is a possibility that this therapy will delay the onset of the disease, and therefore the life-threatening complications.

IGF-I treatment

Unlike the other two therapies, this is a treatment currently being tested after the onset of diabetes. It has been known for some time that people with insulin-dependent diabetes have high levels of growth hormone (which has anti-insulin actions) and low levels of IGF-I, a hormone which has insulin-like metabolic properties. By restoring IGF-I levels it is thought that the high levels of growth hormone secretions might be prevented, which may help stabilize the metabolism and improve control, thus reducing insulin requirements and helping to prevent future complications. Trials are underway in Oxford, England, with adults and adolescents.

Chapter Six

Complementary therapies

Complementary therapies can help many of the problems associated with having diabetes in the family. These therapies treat your child holistically, taking personality as well as the diabetes into account. Children generally respond very well to all forms of natural healing – they have enormous powers for self-healing, and complementary therapies can assist this natural process.

There are many therapies suitable for children which have been shown to help improve the uptake of insulin and encourage good blood sugar control. Others are useful for overcoming particular problems such as needle phobia or acute anxiety. Complementary therapies in general also help children to relax and gain confidence, and to accept and deal with their condition.

Meditation, yoga, acupuncture and massage can all help alleviate stress and anxiety, and a weekly session could become a useful refuge from the daily routines and regimes associated with diabetes. Parents need no special skills to massage their babies or toddlers other than an ability to smooth and stroke their skin gently with a few drops of essential oil added to a sweet-smelling base of apricot oil, a combination which will work perfectly to soothe and restore any fractious child.

And do not forget that these therapies will help parents, too, as suggested in Chapter Three. Being relaxed and in control of your own physical and mental health will empower you and promote inner strength to tackle the 24-hour job of caring for your child.

Used with children complementary therapies can help to counter stress, and treat their overall physical condition and level of wellbeing. In the management of diabetes they do this by:

- eliminating psychological strain through relaxation
- helping to identify behaviour and habits that put the child at risk of unnecessary swings in blood glucose
- stimulating the body's inner healing powers
- toning up tissues and organs, maximizing their full potential
- improving circulation and stabilizing glucose levels in the blood

Natural therapies useful for diabetes

Body and Mind

- aromatherapy
- reflexology
- homeopathy
- cellatroniks and bioresonance therapy
- massage
- naturopathy
- yoga
- meditation
- flower remedies
- acupressure
- healing
- traditional Chinese medicine
- Ayurvedic medicine
- polarity therapy

Emotions

- hypnotherapy
- massage
- relaxation techniques
- counselling

These therapies are of enormous help in assisting the body's own healing process, helping to eliminate toxins and viruses from the body and opening up 'energy channels', sorting out vitamin, mineral or enzyme deficiencies to boost the body's immune system, and strengthening specific organs such as the pancreas.

Note: Reducing stress can help improve control of blood glucose levels but no complementary therapy can replace insulin. No one should be encouraged to reduce insulin or change their children's prescribed dose without advice from a medical consultant. Use complementary therapies as just that – to complement and enhance your lives.

WHY CHOOSE NATURAL THERAPIES?

There will be times when extra help is needed to maintain blood sugar levels – to relieve stress or alleviate the pain and discomfort of injections. You will of course follow the conventional prescribed treatment to ensure that your child can live a symptomless life, but you may feel there is something lacking in this purely conventional approach. You may want something that will support your child's health and immune system. Many families with children with diabetes are therefore turning to complementary therapies for an answer.

Conventional medicine cannot cure diabetes, and the cause is still unknown. This has been the situation for the past 70 years and there is still very little new information about the disease available for parents, in terms of practical care. The only orthodox solution is to keep on taking insulin; there is nothing else that can be done.

But complementary therapies offer another course of action. They give you the opportunity to help your child by strengthening the body, ridding the system of toxins and maximizing an inner sense of wellbeing. None offers a cure, but children will benefit from the restorative effects, which will in turn keep them healthier, both mentally and physically, in the future, when they may be at risk of some of the more unpleasant long-term complications of diabetes.

Natural therapies are based on the belief that the body has an in-built method of healing and supporting itself. Therapies which are suitable for children will help to support their young bodies to meet the challenges that will face them years from now. All those discussed here are safe, and their use may result in some alteration to the insulin dose your child receives. If you do notice this effect consult your medical practitioner.

The therapies can be safely used in conjunction with conventional treatment, although you may want to talk to your practitioner about the therapy you choose before you begin. Many orthodox doctors are now happy to accept that families want to explore complementary therapies, and will welcome your ideas.

A natural therapist will want to meet your child, discuss your lifestyle as a family, and find out about your child's general emotional state. The aim is to restore harmony in the mind and emotions as well as the body, for true healing can only take place when the whole person is treated.

One of the greatest advantages of natural medicine is the close relationship that is established between therapist and patient. In this case the relationship will undoubtedly extend to you as parents. So many parents have complained about the lack of continuity they face at conventional clinics, and the feeling of desperation in having to explain the state of their child's health yet again to another new doctor. With a natural therapist a relationship is built up on a one-to-one basis, which adds an important element of safety and security, especially for children.

While conventional remedies control a disease like diabetes, complementary or natural therapies try and channel it by using the body's natural healing abilities. Moreover, natural therapies are mostly pleasant and positive, with no harmful side-effects.

AROMATHERAPY

Aromatherapy is the use of essential oils to enhance health. Children with diabetes will benefit from the enjoyable smells of different oils, as well as their therapeutic effects. Inhaling essential oils stimulates the part of the brain connected with hormone control, instinctive behaviour and strong emotions.

Aromatherapy has been around for more than 5,000 years, but it was revived this century by a French physician, Dr Jean Valkne, who used essential oils from plants, barks, petals, wood and spices to treat diabetes, amongst other chronic conditions, after the First World War. Today aromatherapy is an accepted part of the conventional medical scene in France.

Care must be taken when using essential oils for children. Only very small amounts should be used – one drop per two stone of body weight. The best way of using them is to put one or two drops of the chosen oil into a bath, although this is not recommended for babies and very tiny children.

Another way of using aromatherapy, which *is* suitable for babies, is to apply two or three drops of an essential oil to a tissue and place it near the cot; one mother uses lavender oil only in the nursery and her baby now associates this soothing scent with sleep and rest. A single drop of oil on nightwear is another way of offering aromatherapy to a young child.

Other ways of administering oils:

- placing a burner in a baby's bedroom – but ensure it is positioned somewhere very safe, and on a solid, firm base, out of reach of small hands
- combining them with a base oil and massaging on to the skin – babies and toddlers love massage in a comfortable warm environment, and giving massage is also relaxing

Suggested oils for diabetes

Lavender is calming and soothing with anti-bacterial and anti-inflammatory properties. **Roman camomile**, distilled from the flowers of *Anthemis nobilis*, is mild and sweet-smelling, and particularly suitable for children. It calms nervousness, aids the digestive system and stimulates white cell production, which is useful when treating infections. It will also help your child get a good night's sleep. Children will love the sweet, rich smell of **mandarin** and it is lovely in a bath or to scent a room. In France it is known as the children's therapy as it is completely non-toxic and has a calming and soothing effect. It is beneficial in the treatment of stress and for uplifting a child's mood. **Geranium** is calming and cooling with an uplifting and strengthening effect, making it useful for alleviating anxiety. **Juniper** is a useful oil for treating teenagers going through puberty, as it helps to promote hormone balance. It is stimulating and astringent and helps the body to remove impurities. On a psychological note, using juniper promotes a more optimistic outlook.

Other useful oils include:

- bergamot, marjoram and rosemary for pain relief
- neroli, tea tree and lavender for cell regeneration
- garlic, lavender and rosewood to boost the immune system
- myrrh, rose, basil, birch, lavender, black pepper and marjoram as general tonics

Buy oils at a reputable shop – cheap oils are virtually useless. If in doubt consult a medical aromatherapist. Remember that essential oils are powerful, so they must always be very well diluted. Never allow your child to swallow them.

Case Study

I massaged my baby with oils from an early age. It was not only relaxing for him, but also for me. He loved the massage, and it helped soothe and settle him and helped rid us both of tension.
Veronica, mother of Benjamin, aged 16

REFLEXOLOGY

Some people describe reflexology as foot massage, but it is more than that. It is based on an ancient therapy and probably has links with acupressure and acupuncture. It is based on the principle that the feet have different zones, which correspond to different parts of the body. Reflexologists use the feet as 'maps' which enable them to assess the whole body's state of health and wellbeing. By applying pressure to particular zones, energy channels in the corresponding parts of the body become unblocked and restored, body toxins are eliminated and circulation is improved. Reflexology does not claim to be able to remove infection or disease but it is certain that treatment can help to alleviate illness.

With a child with diabetes a reflexologist may want to work the area associated with the pancreas, which sits in the centre of the arch of the left foot, rising to join an area associated with the spleen. On the right foot there is a smaller area lying above the part connected to the stomach. The reflexologist will want to feel for areas of blockage and work them to eliminate toxins and stimulate any remaining beta-cells left in the pancreas. The feet are supported firmly but gently as the reflexologist works, so there is no danger of your child bursting into a fit of giggles because the feet are being 'tickled'. Firm, gentle stroking movements are part of the process.

Reflexology will promote a feeling of wellbeing, which will be noticeable immediately after a session. It will help improve a sluggish circulation but above all it is wonderfully relaxing, perfectly safe and suitable for very young children.

Morrell reflexology

Devised by Patricia Morrell this form of reflexology follows different philosophies and different methods. Using feather-light finger pressure practitioners use similar zones on the feet. They begin by blowing warm breath on to the soles of the feet and then use a very light touch to work on them. Sessions for children last between three and five minutes, and are most beneficial for anxious youngsters. They report great success with endocrine problems, bowel cancer and kidney complaints, especially in children.

HOMEOPATHY

Homeopathic treatments can be usefully prescribed for overall health and wellbeing, for specific ailments or for removing viruses and their effects from the body. As mentioned in Chapter Two, some scientists believe that a dormant virus may act as a trigger for Type I diabetes so, if your child suffered from any of the viruses listed on page 17, ask a homeopath for a cleansing treatment, or for one specifically for that virus.

Homeopathic treatments follow the 200-year-old principle established by Samuel Hahnemann, a German doctor, that 'like cures like'. Very small amounts of substance made from a variety of sources – animal, vegetable and mineral – form a solution, which is diluted and then vigorously shaken. The belief is that the more dilute the solution and the more it is shaken, a technique called 'succussion', the more potent is its ability to stimulate the body's own healing powers.

Homeopathic remedies can also help when your child is ill with an infection which healthy children might take in their stride. Antibiotics are sometimes vital, but there has been a lot of debate over how appropriate it is to routinely give children these strong medications, which also kill 'good' bacteria in the gut. Homeopathic remedies are gentle and soothing on body systems, and are an excellent alternative for a child with diabetes, where the aim should be to promote wellbeing and do all you can to support the healthy body systems.

Seek a consultation, as homeopathic remedies work best when they are tailor-made to the individual child. A homeopath will take a personal history and use information about a child's characteristics when preparing a constitutional prescription.

Homeopathic remedies can work very well; they are gentle, soothing and entirely natural, and are appropriate for children already suffering from diabetes. Moreover, there are no side-effects.

Homeopathic preparations suitable for diabetes include:

- nat sulp, silicea and argent nit for the general constitution
- uranium nit for weakness, bedwetting and digestive upsets
- codeinum for restlessness and skin irritation

Homeopathic remedies will help to make the body more responsive to illness by strengthening the immune system and supporting the white blood cells which fight infection. In creating a constitutional remedy for your child with diabetes the homeopath will be looking at ways to support the body systems and offering remedies which will strengthen any weaknesses. Use homeopathic remedies generally for:

- stress and anxiety
- feverish colds, sore throats and headaches
- indigestion
- kidney disorders
- hyperactivity
- bruising on injection sites – try rubbing on some arnica cream

CELLATRONIKS AND BIORESONANCE THERAPY

Cellatroniks is a brand new therapy in the United Kingdom, although it has been practised in the United States for 25 years by its founder Teddy Gagnan. Also called dynamic energy therapy, it boosts energy fields in the body, which in turn strengthens the immune system and enhances the body's healing capacity.

The therapy works by sending invisible and soundless energy waves into the body via key points – the hands, feet, back of the neck, chest, shoulder and abdomen. A central machine stores different programmes for enhancing different parts of the body or body systems – for example, there are programmes for the kidneys, the endocrine system, the digestion, the eyes, the legs and the circulation.

Patients sit in a comfortable chair and the energy is fed into the body via a flat metal plate known as an enhancer. Some patients feel a warmth spreading from the plate, others say they feel no sensation. Laboratory tests have shown that once the energy is passed into the body differences can be found in the brain waves; patients report feeling relaxed and later energized. Teddy Gagnan describes the treatment as 'a food for the body', supplying energy where it is deficient. This in turns helps to achieve balance in the body, enabling it to combat disease and disorder. Cellatroniks technology is currently being used to treat cancer, MS and diabetes in the United States.

Bioresonance therapy is another therapy which works work on the body's own ultrafine electromagnetic oscillations or signals. A machine called the Bicom tunes into the electromagnetic frequencies, some of which are strong and healthy and are called 'harmonic' and others of which are out of balance and called 'disharmonic'. The machine is able to give a read-out of your child's state of health, and where disharmony is detected it amplifies the harmonic or good waves in an attempt to restore balance.

The principle behind the therapy is that the electromagnetic signals which emanate from all living things are disturbed by illness. By restoring their flow, the body is able to start to heal itself. Therapists are willing to treat children with diabetes to boost the immune system and to help restore cell function in a failing pancreas.

MASSAGE

Massaging your baby or very young child with gentle stroking movements and maybe some sweet-smelling and soothing oils will help promote a feeling of love and security, as well as general health and happiness. Touch is one of the most natural processes in the world and is an expression of love and safety. Children and babies benefit enormously from massage – babies are found to gain weight and young children become less anxious.

Touching plays a major role in child development and massage can coax tension from muscles and improve blood circulation. It is good for babies who have colic or cry at night. It will also help negative emotional feelings and encourage a sense of self-worth and self-esteem. It will stimulate the flow of blood throughout the body, and above all make your child feel loved and well cared for, even though she is living with a daily routine of injections and may carry more psychological burdens and responsibilities than other children of the same age.

There are different forms of massage. Children may respond particularly well to effleurage, a system of simple, light touching or stroking and knuckling which can be used with a deep or light pressure and has the ability to increase the flow of blood to a specific part of the body.

NATUROPATHY

The basic principle of naturopathy is that the body has the ability to heal itself. It focuses on stimulating the body's own vital force using these principles:

- clean air and water
- organic food
- exercise and healthy living

Naturopaths are often trained in a range of skills which include herbalism, homeopathy, massage and nutrition and diet. The aim is to restore health and vitality by looking after the body in the way nature intended. Naturopaths believe that disease occurs when the body is thrown out of balance by the environment, genetic influence and destructive emotions – feelings such as hate or stress for example can upset hormone balance. This ties in perfectly with what the orthodox scientists believe are the trigger factors of diabetes.

Around the world there is a growing recognition of natural medicine, with the underlying belief that infections rarely take hold in bodies which are well cared for and well maintained. But naturopathy requires commitment from those receiving the treatment, and may call for whole changes to one's lifestyle.

Dietary and nutritional advice will help all families with children with diabetes. A naturopath may recommend supplementing your child's diet with magnesium and chromium, which are important for the uptake of insulin and glucose tolerance in the body. Herbal medicine may also be recommended. And although fasting, which is often used as a means of cleansing the body, is not appropriate for children with diabetes, the principles of healthy living can certainly be adopted, and will undoubtedly boost the immune system, which in turn will help the body to fight off infections more readily and keep blood glucose levels more stable.

Naturopaths take into account the whole child and are interested in the psychological significance of stress. They also like to encourage their patients to make changes to their lives, which result in healthier living.

YOGA

Children as young as six can benefit from yoga exercises, which not only work on the physical body but also relax the mind, help children to concentrate and relax, and teach them to be quiet and still. Yoga can help children:

- regain the flexibility and suppleness they had as babies
- remain calm if they feel stressed
- come to terms with the pressures of adolescence
- understand more about their bodies and how they work

Robin Munro of the UK Yoga Biomedical Trust reports that research in India has shown some very positive results for people with insulin-dependent diabetes with regard to the control of blood glucose levels.

Yoga therapy promotes the body's own natural healing process by using physical and mental techniques directed at specific ailments and conditions. Children with diabetes will benefit from the way it encourages body control and body awareness. As diabetes is ever present, good body image is vital for your child's self-esteem.

Breathing exercises will be helpful before injections or blood glucose testing. Moreover, if your child is not a 'sporty' type, yoga will help promote fitness and strength in a gentle, non-competitive way.

It can also be great fun, and can involve movements designed to promote good co-ordination. Many yoga poses are based on the natural grace of animals, and are named after the animals they emulate, such as Lion, Mouse, Snake, Butterfly and Cheetah. This may prove inspirational as well as fun for your child.

Contact a teacher with a special interest in teaching yoga to children – they should always be supervised until they know exactly what they are doing. Working in groups also makes the whole exercise pleasurable. To provide a good foundation children should take part in yoga exercises at least once a week.

MEDITATION

The word 'meditation' comes from the Sanskrit word *medha*, meaning wisdom – through meditation we get to know ourselves better. It may seem like a very grown-up thing to do, but children can also benefit from it. However, do not expect young children to be able to concentrate for more than a few minutes at the start.

The long-term benefits of meditation for children with diabetes include a boost in self-confidence and self-esteem. Through meditation, they learn to take more control, and when living with diabetes it is easy to feel 'out of control', trapped in the cycle of food, injections and monitoring.

You can either learn about meditation yourself and then get the whole family involved (read *Teaching Meditation to Children* by David Fontana and Ingrid Slack) or contact a local meditation practitioner and ask whether there are any suitable family classes. Try and encourage a special time for meditating, and choose a quiet room in which to do it away from the distractions of TV and radio. Ensure that your child is relaxed before meditating, and try to increase the length of the meditation each week. Children under five may only be able to participate for two or three minutes, but children aged six to ten should be able to meditate for at least five to ten minutes a day.

FLOWER REMEDIES

Flower remedies are restorative and enjoyable, dealing with negative emotions by balancing energies and encouraging an enhanced sense of wellbeing. They are useful for treating moods and the state of mind.

The remedies are made from the flowers of wild plants, bushes and trees. The best known are the Bach Flower Remedies named after the British homeopath, Dr Edward Bach, who created an original range of 39 remedies in the 1920s and 1930s. Other remedies are made throughout the world.

It is useful to match your child's personality with an appropriate flower remedy, as each has its own characteristics. For children with diabetes try **honeysuckle**, which helps put the past in perspective, and **cherry plum** to deal with inner turmoil. **Cerato** will enable your child to trust her own judgement while **crab apple** is good for young people going through the turmoil of puberty, **mimulus** helps develop courage and **red chestnut** helps put fears into perspective. **Bach's Rescue Remedy** is useful for reduce the after-effects of shock and trauma and stimulating the healing powers of the body. It helps in emergencies when your child feels panicky or shocked and will be a useful remedy to keep at home to deal with the after-effects of a hypo.

Flower remedies are completely safe and no contra-indications have been reported.

ACUPRESSURE

If you feel your child has enough of needles in everyday life, acupressure may be an alternative to acupuncture. It is often called acupuncture without needles, and indeed some people believe it may have been an early form of acupuncture.

There are a number of variations, perhaps the best known being shiatsu. This is a Japanese word meaning finger pressure – acupressure uses finger pressure, sometimes elbow, knee or heel pressure, on the same points of the body as acupuncture. The principles behind acupressure are the same as those behind acupuncture in that it is believed to stimulate the energy lines or meridians to promote the flow of chi (pronounced *chee*) or life force, and may help to stimulate the hormonal system in the case of children with diabetes.

HEALING

People often refer to this as 'faith healing', and it involves nothing more than the touch or thoughts of the practitioner. Healing energy is somehow passed through the hands of a healer to the recipient, and it works on the body as well as the mind. It is thought that a healer acts as a channel for some outside force or energy which has the ability to stimulate the body's own healing powers. Some healers concentrate on the chakras, the seven main energy centres of the body, concentrating on a particular centre, depending on the ailment being helped.

Therapeutic touch or TT, as it is known in the United States, is also based on the belief that there is a transfer of energy between healer and recipient, and it is commonly found in hospitals across the United States.

TRADITIONAL CHINESE MEDICINE (TCM)

TCM is based on the underlying principle of yin and yang, the opposing energies in the universe, which must be in harmony within us. It involves a combination of herbal medicine and acupuncture to help restore balance and involves a complicated diagnostic system that includes examining the tongue, ears, face, hands and feet. Dietary advice will be offered, which may be very helpful for children with diabetes.

Diabetes may be considered a kidney/spleen imbalance, and herbs might be prescribed to nourish weak organs and generally strengthen the body. British researchers have been looking at herbal remedies for diabetes found throughout the world and have found that xiaoke tea, an infusion of dried leaves, has the ability to lower blood glucose levels.

AYURVEDIC MEDICINE

This is the main form of traditional medicine found in India and is often described as one of the most complete systems of natural health care found anywhere in the world. The system involves 20 different approaches to health through mind, body, behaviour and environment. Much emphasis is placed on nutrition, lifestyle, environment and emotions.

There are some 8,000 different herbal medicines available in the system, but apart from this the main emphasis is on changing lifestyle and diet which, interestingly, is also the Western approach to managing Type I diabetes. The content and preparation of food are considered important (also part of a Western approach to diabetes), and it is believed that certain foods can reduce anxiety while others increase energy levels.

This form of medicine is safe in qualified hands. A responsible practitioner will never ask you to give up your child's conventional treatment but will merely adapt the therapy. Many herbal medicines are useful for controlling blood sugar levels, but this has

to be weighed against the daily dosage of insulin prescribed for
your child.

■ POLARITY THERAPY

This therapy took 50 years to develop and was born out of a study
of Eastern practices, mysticism and ancient forms of medicine
such as Ayurvedic and yoga. The aim is to balance opposing
energies in the body by aligning mental, physical and emotional
health.

The founder of polarity therapy, Dr Randolph Stone, a
naturopath from Chicago, saw the body as a living magnet with
electromagnetic energy flowing between positive and negative
poles. Disease, he believed, was the result of energy trapped by
poor diet and a lack of energy.

Using the system of chakras as the points from which
energy flows, polarity therapy aims to release trapped energy, thus
enabling the body to heal itself. This can be done through
attention to diet, yoga-type exercises, massage techniques and
counselling. Children with diabetes may benefit from its energy-
boosting techniques and from the specific dietary advice.

A calm interior (the mind) can influence the exterior (the body).
Inner turmoil can affect diabetes because of the impact the stress
hormones have on blood glucose levels, causing high or low
swings. As we have seen (*see* Chapter Two), there is evidence
that stressful life events such as parents separating or any other
major trauma can actually speed up the attack by antibodies on
the insulin-producing cells, triggering an early onset of the
disease. The following therapies will help to overcome stress and
promote calmness of mind.

HYPNOTHERAPY

In the hands of a qualified practitioner the art of hypnotherapy is quite safe, but ensure you track down a reputable therapist. It is a powerful therapy, but do not worry about someone trying to force you or your child into doing things you do not want to do – most hypnotherapists use a light trance which simply makes patients susceptible to what is being said. It is not advisable for children under the age of five, however.

Hypnotherapy can help children with diabetes to:

- overcome any fears or anxieties about their condition
- overcome feelings of pain when injecting or testing blood glucose levels

It will also benefit parents if they have underlying feelings of guilt or self-blame.

A hypnotherapist might want to take between four and five sessions to address a particular problem. As hypnotherapy goes directly to the subconscious mind, problems may be resolved more quickly than by going to a conventional counsellor. One area of success is in treating children who have a fear of needles or feel pain at injection time. A useful technique, which can be easily taught to a receptive child, is the ability to create a 'magic finger', which will not feel pain at blood-test time.

MASSAGE

Massage can be wonderfully therapeutic for children, as it engenders a sense of safety and love. It can be calming and beneficial for children who are beset by worries about their diabetes, or who realize for the first time that it will be there for every day of their life. Younger children respond well to massage before they become too 'body aware'. Teenagers may need more encouragement but, if they have grown up with parents who touch and hug automatically, then massage will not be an alien concept.

RELAXATION TECHNIQUES

Relaxation may help your child's diabetes, as it restores an inner sense of peace and harmony. It may help older children cope with feelings of resentment, anger or envy at not being the same as their schoolfriends, and always having to be careful about food, drink and lifestyle.

For an older child the technique may be something as simple as a cup of camomile tea and being tucked up in a warm bed with a hot water bottle and a teddy bear. The aim is to help your child banish negative feelings and replace 'bad' thoughts with 'good' ones. Relaxation tapes may help encourage sleep. Children can also be taught to identify tension in muscles and to relax them by going through the parts of the body and encouraging them to 'go floppy'. This will help your child understand what it means to relax, and to feel the difference between a tense muscle and a relaxed one.

COUNSELLING

Counselling is explained in detail in Chapter Three (*see* pages 35–7). It can help children to explore problems and clarify them, and to lay to rest fears about diabetes. It is useful if they are beset by worries about their condition, or if they are suffering from depression. (Children do suffer from depression, just like adults, although it may be more difficult to detect. Warning signs are withdrawal and behavioural problems.)

Counsellors have the skills to listen to your child and convey warmth and interest. You may find it helpful to visit someone with a close association with diabetes, or you may consider family therapy, when the whole family attends for counselling sessions.

Counselling can empower you and your child, and help you to manage the diabetes more easily if there are problems. Counsellors will encourage your child to learn more about the disorder and accept it as part of herself. Several sessions will probably be necessary in order to reap the full benefit.

Chapter Seven

As they grow: under fives

A quarter of all cases of insulin-dependent diabetes are diagnosed before the child's fifth birthday, only a tiny percentage are babies under the age of two.

When diabetes is diagnosed this early in life parents are bound to experience feelings of fear and anguish. In many ways it is the parents who are in need of tender, loving care. Having just celebrated the arrival of a perfect infant, they are told a few months or years later that the child has a serious, life-threatening condition. Parents often say, with hindsight, that their child took diabetes in his stride; it was *their* emotions that were the problem. A child diagnosed with diabetes as an infant will remember no other state, but will pick up any anxieties or fears you show. It is therefore important to find a way of coping that suits you and your baby – but the key to your new lifestyle will be flexibility. You will find that no sooner have you addressed one stage than another will emerge to challenge you! But in many respects this reflects the delights and difficulties of parenting in general.

But there are many practical worries connected with looking after a baby or toddler with diabetes. How can a two-year-old possibly understand why it is so important to have this snack, or that injection? Infants respond to warmth, care and love, and they begin developing trust. But children diagnosed with diabetes at this early stage may be faced with painful procedures and stressful encounters with strangers in the form of the medical and nursing team. It is at these times that massage and aromatherapy can be useful to provide a soothing atmosphere. If your baby associates the smell of lavender oil with your bedtime routine, for example, then carry this on if he has to be admitted to hospital. Routines help promote feelings of security so carry on with as many as possible – in the mornings, at mealtimes, when it is time for a nap and at bedtime.

Hospitals nowadays encourage parents to stay with their children as more is understood about separation anxiety, which is most acute between six months and four years of age. Infants need to build up trust in those around them even if they associate a carer with the pain of an injection.

Toddlers meanwhile will start to develop a sense of their own identity, and become more independent. There will be a balancing act between giving your child a first taste of independence and being overprotective.

Talking about diabetes will help your child accept the illness from an early stage. Reassurance is essential, as some children can develop feelings of shame or guilt and see their disease as a punishment. A further danger at this stage is the transfer of guilt or stress from the parents on to the child through anxiety or overindulgence, or by being too strict with eating regimes and injections.

Praise your child and do not punish lapses. Try and focus on the positive, on 'getting it right for tomorrow'. But children can be manipulative and may demand rewards for sticking to the insulin regime, which is a tricky cycle to escape from. Adapt your routines to take account of what is planned during the day.

Case Study

Bringing our child home from hospital after a diagnosis of diabetes was just like bringing a new baby back into the home. It was traumatic and disturbing, as we had a new way of life in front of us. It was just like starting afresh.

Jayne, mother of Debbie, aged two

Special note: Insulin-dependent diabetes is rare in children under the age of six months. However there is a condition called neonatal or transient diabetes which most often occurs in infants under the age of six weeks who are usually born small for their gestational age. The symptoms include vomiting, diarrhoea and rapid weight loss. This form of diabetes usually disappears after a few weeks, although some of these babies may develop Type I diabetes later in life.

THE BIRTH FACTOR

Australian researchers have suggested that a diabetic child's birth weight and development in the womb may influence the age at which Type I diabetes is diagnosed in a susceptible child. Smaller babies (under 2.5kg) showed a 'significantly' earlier onset of diabetes (between the ages of three and six). A study took into account birth weights, length, gestational age, weight at six months and feeding history during the first six months of life. Predicting early onset could become an important factor in deciding when intervention therapies might be given.

BREAST FEEDING

Breast feeding not only gives babies the right start in life, but may also help to boost their immunity to a number of ailments. Breast feeding a child with diabetes is ideal, as babies feed often, including during the night.

Babies with diabetes are able to follow the same weaning pattern as any other infants. Solids such as fruit purées and rice-based cereals can be introduced from three months of age, but if you can, stick with breast feeding as part of your baby's diet for the first year of your baby's life.

Once your baby starts to sleep through the night you will probably need to adjust the insulin dose to prevent night-time hypos. Regular mealtimes should be introduced from the start to help encourage good glucose control, although every parent will understand that the often chaotic lives of infants and toddlers means that this is not always possible.

DIET

Toddlers tend to be on the go from morning to night, and need energy-dense foods. A small amount of food every two hours will help to maintain blood sugar levels. Toddlers usually respond well to routine, so take full advantage of this. Research in the United States has shown that high-carbohydrate foods combined with foods high in soluble fibre (such as beans) help to lower blood glucose levels in children with diabetes. However you should be careful about giving a very young child large amounts of fibre – overdosing can lead to poor absorption of essential minerals and vitamins.

Foods which will help control blood sugars include lentils, pulses, peas and porridge. An ideal lunch for a hungry toddler could well be something as simple as lentil burgers and wholemeal bread. Keep plenty of wholesome snacks readily at hand – for example sliced hard boiled eggs, fresh fruit, sticks of organic carrots, wholemeal bread and low-salt organic peanut butter. Introduce semi-skimmed milk from the age of two.

Strive to reduce sugar in the diet by:

- baking cakes with wholemeal flour and either fruit such as dates or half the amount of sugar suggested
- buying reduced sugar jams or spreads
- sweetening home-made puddings with fruit – but make puddings a treat and substitute fresh fruit or a low-fat fruit yoghurt.

Parties and treats

Most toddlers have a flourishing social life with invitations to tea or lunch. Don't let your child miss out on these treats even though you may feel nervous at the prospect at first. You may wish to increase the dose of insulin by a very small amount to give extra cover if you know your child is going to be faced with an irresistible array of undesirable food.

Don't deprive your child of a slice of cake at a party, but be flexible about food intake and insulin requirements on that day, taking into account the fact that there are bound to be more high-fat carbohydrate foods at the party than usual. Encourage him to opt for sandwiches rather than sweets, and save any sweets he brings home in a special jar which can be used for exceptional treats.

Fat

Children under two and toddlers need extra energy for growth and play. Don't cut back on fat in the diet before the age of two, but after that gradually switch to a lower-fat diet (such as exchanging full-fat milk to semi-skimmed, and using low-fat yoghurts). It should be mentioned that there are some people who believe it better to continue with 'whole milk' until a later age, and reduce fat in other foods in the diet. Fat in milk contains the Vitamin D required for the absorption of calcium.

Fussy eating

It is quite common for small children to be fussy eaters and it can be quite worrying. Food can become an even greater battle-ground between parents and a child with diabetes because of the importance it has in their daily welfare.

If your toddler is going through a fussy eating phase stress and tension may well surround meal times. Although you may feel desperate that your child is only eating two or three different foods, or simply will not eat, be reassured that this is only a temporary phase.

In the meantime you could try:

- offering small amounts of food at a time, as your child can always come back for more – little and often may become your guide during this difficult patch, and you could try for 20g of carbohydrate at each meal with 20g of snacks
- making mealtimes enjoyable by eating together and praising your child when he eats up
- coaxing rather than forcing your child to eat, and just taking the plate away and giving a drink containing carcohydrate like a glass of milk – be flexible, not forceful
- establishing a routine, and being careful that your child does not fill up too much on drinks
- making a list of all the foods your child enjoys and offering these most often
- working together with your partner to form a united front so that your child learns to understand that there is a routine to mealtimes
- making a special effort to encourage your child to eat breakfast
- trying to compromise, and appreciating what your child will and will not eat – make a list of his favourite foods and every so often add new foods
- allowing your child to help prepare the food
- using fun plates to make mealtimes more attractive
- having a pretend picnic on the floor if things become difficult
- allowing your child to watch TV while eating if necessary.

Case Study

My advice to parents is to keep expectations low about the food your toddler is going to eat – give small amounts at first, then he can always come back for more. Be prepared to sit down on the floor and play games, use toys such as plastic cups and saucers, and pastry cutters to make shapes with bread, and use the TV as a distraction if necessary. Get your child involved in mealtimes but above all make it fun, make it pleasurable and get your child interested in choosing what he wants to eat. If he refuses something one day, then go back to it again a few days later.

Christine, mother of Sean, aged five

■ AVOIDING BABY 'BURN-OUT'

You should try to give yourself a break from your baby from time to time. It might be difficult to find someone to take over for a while, as you have to feel confident that you can trust them, and you will have to educate them about your child's illness. But it is important to allow yourself a break from the daily pressures. You do not want to become exhausted or isolated, and an occasional day off from the 24-hour care of your child is important for your own wellbeing. Moreover, when a baby has diabetes the nurturing role is heightened and there is a real risk of the child becoming overdependent. Babies need to learn that they can be safe and content without their parents for short spells, so try and find the support of someone close to you who will be happy to take over the care of your child. You could start with just a short break – perhaps an hour – and gradually extend the time as you and the carer gain confidence in the arrangement.

■ INJECTIONS

If the same injection site is used too often it can become lumpy and the insulin will not work properly, so it is important to change the site from time to time. The main injection sites are:

- the front and outside of the thighs
- the stomach
- the buttocks

Insulin is absorbed most rapidly:

- from a subcutaneous injection over the abdomen
- from the arm rather than the leg
- after a hot bath

However a rapid reaction is not always desirable.

If a spot becomes sore, try using arnica cream on it. Other useful treatments for bruising include using a natural beeswax cream with added rose water, sweet almond oil and lavender oil to ease swelling and pain and encourage internal healing. Or you could try a compress of rosemary to encourage circulation.

You will be told at diagnosis how many units of insulin your child needs. Your baby will grow quickly and the insulin requirements will change, so expect to visit your diabetes specialist at least once every two or three months for an update. You will get instruction on how to inject your baby, and will be equipped with special fine needles to help you with the job. The best syringes for babies are low-dose disposable ones. Keep the insulin at room temperature to make it more comfortable as it goes into the bloodstream. The way you give the injection is important – your baby will pick up anxiety, tension and fear and can be upset by these negative emotions. Take turns with a partner or another close relative so that it is not just one person's job.

■ HOLIDAYS

When flying, carry your child's diabetes equipment in your hand luggage, and keep it with you at all times. Do not allow it to go into the hold of the aircraft in your main luggage as it could very well get lost, and even if it does not the insulin could freeze. Be prepared for delays, and if your child is fully weaned take extra food and snacks, also in your hand luggage. Take double the amount of insulin you will need in case of broken bottles, and store it in a wide-necked thermos packed with ice if you are visiting a hot country. Do not forget the extra supplies of sugar-free drinks.

Be careful in a hot climate as sunburn – or even simply heat – can affect blood sugar levels. Climate changes may also affect your child's insulin requirements, so watch out for any changes in reaction to the normal dose. Also ask your doctor for a letter confirming your child's condition, and if you are going abroad have it translated into the local language.

You do not want the added complication of your child suffering from travel sickness, if it can be avoided. Try a wristband which presses on the acupressure point on the wrist and which can alleviate motion sickness. Or dab a few drops of ginger oil on a tissue for your child to sniff. A homeopath may offer tabacum for nausea.

ILLNESS

Your child will be just as likely as any other child to catch coughs, colds and other infections such as chicken pox and measles. If there is an illness going around at playgroup there is no point in keeping your child away – it will only reinforce any feelings of being different. The infections which cause parents of children with diabetes the most concern are stomach upsets with vomiting and diarrhoea.

When your child becomes ill blood glucose levels will tend to rise, although in some children they do fall initially due to the change in the metabolic rate caused by the infection or due to food not being kept down. The change in blood sugar levels is the body's response to an infection. As the immune system sets to work to destroy the bug, adrenalin is released, as well as glucose, to fuel the fight. It is vital to carry on giving insulin just as before. If there is not enough insulin fat will be broken down for energy, and ketones, which are produced if the body needs insulin, will be released, and may start to appear in the urine if blood sugar levels stay at over 17 mmol/l for two to five hours or longer. Ketones may cause stomach cramps and then vomiting, and if this happens your child will need to go to hospital.

If your child becomes ill:

- do not stop giving insulin
- try to get your child to eat some carbohydrate
- make sure his urine is tested for signs of ketones
- carry out blood glucose checks every two hours or so to monitor how your child is reacting to the illness
- replace food with a sugary drink if your child won't eat, in order to maintain glucose levels in the blood
- offer plenty of plain water – drinking will help dilute blood glucose
- give an extra small dose of insulin if blood sugars rise too high

To clear infection from the system avoid mucus-forming dairy products, and offer foods with plenty of crushed garlic or leek, which also act as blood glucose lowering agents. You can also try complementary therapies such as homeopathy (*see* Chapter Six).

Thrush

Children with diabetes may suffer from bouts of thrush if glucose levels are too high. It may show as redness and itching, with a white curd-like discharge. A drop of anti-fungal tea tree oil in an oil base is a useful remedy for this troublesome condition.

Immunization

Your child should have all the usual vaccinations that any other child would expect to receive, at the appropriate age. Ask your doctor about having a flu jab once a year to protect against this annual, changing virus or ask your homeopath about homeopathic immunization, which can help the body to improve its immune response.

▓ STARTING PLAYGROUP

Case Study
At first I was terrified at letting my child out of my sight. But she loves going to playgroup now, and the organizers have adapted the playgroup around her snack times – each child gets a drink of milk and a biscuit at 10.30 am, so that she does not feel different from the others.

Marion, mother of Elaine, aged four

There is no reason why children with diabetes should not join a playgroup like any other two- or three-year-olds. Make an appointment to discuss your child's condition with the playgroup leaders, and ensure they have a contact telephone number. Your child will need to be able to eat a mid-morning snack, but you will probably find the playgroup flexible. Attending playgroup encourages children with diabetes to start thinking about their condition and its requirements, and is an important stepping stone towards full-time schooling.

Chapter Eight

Middle childhood and school

Every diabetic must realise that his health lies mainly in his own hands.

Dr Robin Lawrence, *The Diabetic Life*, 1925

During middle childhood, between the ages of 6 and 12, there is a great enthusiasm for work, and sense of pride in doing well. Children become more involved with friends of the same age, separate from parents more easily and quickly acquire mental, physical and social skills.

PSYCHOLOGICAL DEVELOPMENT

There are several hurdles at this stage of development for children with Type I diabetes – the fear of being different can become acute, especially if school or sports sessions are missed. A different diet, or the need to eat wholesome snacks at set times also sets them apart and there may be clashes with parents over injection regimes. They still need parental supervision but are growing in independence, and their need to do things their way can lead to conflict within the family. During this stage they will become mature enough to start injecting themselves and this will give them some feeling of control over their condition. Books featuring children with diabetes might be helpful in clarifying the fact that there are plenty of other children in the world who have the same condition.

It is at this stage that you need to start transferring responsibility for treatment to your child. By the age of nine children are usually mature enough to inject their own insulin and to understand the need to balance food and energy. However they will still want to security of parental guidance even though they may fight against it furiously! But instead of nagging and scolding, try a reward system. Make a star chart which illustrates what should be done each day; when enough stars are earned give a reward or treat. Praise is still vital when your child does well.

As children start showing signs of wanting to take over some of the responsibility for their own care, it is a good idea to encourage their interest. It will enhance their self-esteem, give them a greater sense of self-worth and help them to accept that diabetes is a vital part of their whole self. Studies have shown that children who take some control over their welfare from an early stage go on to show a greater sense of self-confidence in later years while children with low self-esteem are more likely to experience badly controlled diabetes.

It is important to get in touch with how your child feels about diabetes – talking to each other will help. If you are open, your child will follow suit and will not lapse into secretiveness about the condition. Try and stay calm, and do not over-react to any indiscretions. Teach your child how to be flexible with diabetes care, and show that she can start to make decisions rather than relying on you. Obviously you must still play an important part, but as your child ends primary school education she should be capable of managing most of the daily routine.

■ SPORT

Children of this age will want to take part in regular sporting activities, and this should be actively encouraged. During physical activity the body converts glucose in the blood to energy, which is then used up by the muscles. Before taking part in any physical sporting activity it's important to 'soak up' any excess insulin by having a carbohydrate snack and, if the exercise is continuous and strenuous, your child should have extra carbohydrate at half time.

■ SCHOOL

Starting school is a major milestone in the life of any child, but you may be particularly worried about how your child is going to cope. A full discussion of the implications of diabetes will help both you and your child's teacher feel more confident. The teacher should know some basic facts about diabetes, and in particular about:

- hypos
- the importance of regular meals and snack times
- the importance of an extra carbohydrate snack before sport

The teacher should also be advised never to send your child home alone without notice, and to tell you if there are changes to the school day, such as a delayed mealtime.

Children with diabetes do not like to be made to feel different from their classmates, so teachers should try and ensure that they have as normal a school life as possible, which means being included in all outings, sports events and special days. The aim is not to overprotect them, only to have a small amount of extra care.

There is no reason why your child should not enjoy a full school life – it is fortunate that much of school life is carried on with a routine, so that there will be a morning break for a snack, and possibly an afternoon break. And if you invest in a digital watch with an alarm, it will remind your child – and the teacher – when a mid-morning or afternoon snack is due.

You might well find that the rest of the class is both supportive and helpful to your child. If the class can be told about diabetes, the importance of snacks, injections and even a little about hypos it will help to prevent children's playtime gossip. Later, you could suggest diabetes is chosen as a topic for a science project.

Action you can take to help your child at school

- Fill in a Diabetes Record Card (available in the UK from the British Diabetic Association) with contact telephone numbers, information about hypos and their symptoms, and the treatment. Ensure that everyone who comes into contact with your child – each class teacher – has a copy.
- If most children take a packed lunch then allow your child to do the same. Choose a varied meal plan – wholemeal pitta bread, organic fruit and salads, a tub of brown rice with a dash of olive oil.
- If your child has to stay behind at school for detention or an extra class explain to the teachers that it is vital for your child to be able to have extra food to cover this period.
- Blood sugar levels can rise or fall with stress, so keep an eye on things during the first week at a new school, and later during examinations. It is often a question of trial and error as to how your child will react and cope with stress at school. Yoga and meditation may help to focus your child on her priorities.
- Bullying or picking on your child because of diabetes should be nipped swiftly in the bud. The best weapon is knowledge – if classmates understand why certain children have to have extra snacks, or injections during school hours, they may reduce their playground gossip and accusations.
- Be open with everyone, including other parents, about your child's diabetes. The more people who know about the condition the better. Most people's fears about diabetes are due to a lack of knowledge and information.

There are also questions your child could ask the teacher, such as:

- Can I tell you what happens when I get 'low'?
- How can I let you know when I feel unwell – should I raise my hand?
- Can I do a blood test in the classroom?
- Am I allowed to have a snack during the afternoon lesson?

- Where can I have my injection – do I have to go to another room?

TAKING RESPONSIBILITY

Children as young as six can be encouraged and taught to inject themselves with insulin, although adult supervision will be needed for children of this age. Taking responsibility for their own diabetes care is one of the most important milestones in the lives of children with this condition.

Encourage your child to learn how the insulin is mixed, to wash her hands before injection time, and to see exactly how and where you position the needle for the injection. It is also important for your child to know where you put the used syringes and how to dispose of them safely.

If your child finds injections painful make sure the angle of injection is right and the skin is not being stretched. Use the small needles and syringes that are available, or try the injector pen devices.

DIABETES HOLIDAY CAMPS

These special camps are organized by different diabetes care groups in the United Kingdom and the United States. There are a number of advantages:

- They allow children to meet others with diabetes.
- They give them the confidence to cope on their own without you for a short while.
- They give you a break from the everyday worries of diabetes in the knowledge that your child is in the care of professionals who know and understand everything necessary about diabetes.

The aim of the holiday camps is to provide a relaxed, safe setting for an enjoyable holiday for your child. There will be opportunities to try new sports and maybe learn more about their diabetes. At the camps, doctors and specialist nurses are on hand as well as dietitians, but the atmosphere is relaxed rather than overprotective.

FAMILY HOLIDAYS

Diabetes should not prevent you and your child from going on holiday, even if it involves long-haul travel and a different climate at your destination. Trips abroad – skiing, for example – can prove to you and your child that diabetes need not disqualify your family from enjoying active holidays. But go prepared, and follow the advice in the previous chapter on taking extra supplies and keeping your diabetes kit in your hand luggage (*see* page 89). Order a vegetarian meal on the plane rather than the standard meal, which is usually low in carbohydrate, and ask for extra bread or wholemeal crackers.

As I said in the previous chapter, it is a good idea to take a letter from your diabetes specialist explaining your child's condition, which can be read by customs and immigration officials, and take another in the language of the country you are visiting in case you need to see a doctor while you are away. Take extra care with drinking local water – drink only bottled varieties to be on the safe side – and take all the usual precautions such as vaccinations, malaria tablets, and so on. Take advice from a travel clinic; explain that your child has diabetes and ask about the particular health risks in the country you are travelling to. If your child suffers from travel sickness ask your doctor to prescribe a travel pill to help prevent sickness or try the complementary treatments mentioned on page 90.

A COMPLEMENTARY MEDICINE BOX

Treating your child holistically means investing in natural remedies which are helpful on a day-to-day basis. It can be useful to keep a medicine box of the most common remedies. Other items can be kept in the food store cupboard. The following might form the basis of such a collection:

- for stomach upsets: slippery elm, either in tablet or powder form;
- for nausea and travel sickness: fresh ginger infused and drunk as a tea;
- to boost the immune system: garlic capsules or fresh garlic in food;
- to encourage relaxation and alleviate stress: camomile or the homeopathic preparation rhus tox;
- to alleviate swelling and take away the stinging feeling after injection: lavender oil or witch hazel.

Chapter Nine

The teen years

▥ THE PROBLEMS OF ADOLESCENCE

Adolescence is the period of transition from childhood to adulthood. It is a time of physical and mental growth as well as sexual maturation. Teenagers tend to become sensitive to the way they look and act, and highly aware of all their body changes.

Adolescence is often seen as a stormy period; conflicts arise because of teenagers' need to break away from their parents yet finding, infuriatingly, that they are still very dependent upon them. This can give rise to unpredictable behaviour, veering from the mature to the childish.

Dr Jill Challener, a consultant paediatrician in Cambridgeshire, UK, has made a special study of diabetes and teenagers. She concludes that the condition inevitably affects the normal processes of development – teenagers with diabetes may have delayed sexual and physical maturation and lack self-esteem because of the need for regular check-ups, injections and blood tests. Independence from parents is generally slower in coming because of prolonged parental concern, and teenage battles tend to be fought over diabetes rather than the usual teenage problem areas.

Teenagers with diabetes may also direct their anger towards the health-care team looking after them – it is really their way of fighting back at the disease which marks them out as different from their friends. There may be difficulty accepting all the rules of diabetes care, especially food management and regular injections. Boundaries will be tested to the limit; your child may even ignore all you and others have said about diabetes, especially if he is feeling fine.

Dr Challener's research has shown that teenagers need clear, simple, visual guidance in order for them to appreciate and understand the importance of good control. It is far easier for them to relate to a graph of their blood sugar levels than a number. She believes they need special handling, without abstract notions or warnings about 'the future' but with plenty of practical, sympathetic and above all simple advice on how to maintain their health and promote their independence.

The following chart shows the problems a teenager with diabetes might encounter.

TEENAGERS AND DIABETES

Aims of normal adolescence	How diabetes can interfere
Physical and sexual maturation	Delayed sexual maturation Small stature Invasion of privacy Frequent examinations
Conformity with peer group	Meals must be eaten on time Injections and blood tests
Self-image	Hypos which expose the difference
Self-esteem	Defective body image
Independence from parents	Parental concern Battles over diabetes
Economic independence	Discrimination by employers

▓ HOW TO COPE

Teenagers should be encouraged to enrol in an adolescent clinic. Let them go alone as this reinforces the idea that diabetes is, ultimately, their responsibility and not their parents'. Contact local diabetic groups, which might organize holidays and camps. Be prepared for the worst, and expect a bumpy ride. Your child may change from having a good, reliable attitude to being grumpy and rebellious. Explain that the highs and lows of blood sugar levels are not anyone's 'fault', and that growth hormones are responsible. Go with the flow as your child develops from infant to teenager. It means a shift in the understanding of his needs at each stage of development. Eventually control has to be handed over and there will be a worrying period of 'letting go'. You will have to accept that you cannot watch over a teenager as you can a toddler, but you can still communicate and discuss issues which are important, such as alcohol, drugs and sex.

Introduce your child to the concept of complementary therapies – there is a growing interest among young people in holistic remedies. Suggest yoga, reflexology and aromatherapy.

The most common time for diabetes to be diagnosed is between the ages of 10 and 15, which coincides with puberty, the time of greatest physical upheaval change and growth. But if your child was diagnosed earlier, you will be used to managing the diabetes. During these next few years your main concern will be handing over responsibility. The key to a successful transfer is giving your child enough confidence to manage the condition and make decisions about his wellbeing and welfare.

▓ In summary

- Encourage your teenager to attend a young person's clinic. Find a clinic which will offer clear guidelines for health education, off-clinic activities and a united, sympathetic team of professionals who will reward good control and offer advice during a bad patch (*see* opposite).

- Try not to show too much concern or nag.
- Encourage your child to act as a 'teacher' for a younger child with diabetes.
- Send your teenager to a diabetes camp to mix with other young people of the same age.
- Suggest some of the complementary therapies mentioned earlier.

Teenagers and diabetes

Researchers in Scotland, which has one of the highest rates of insulin-dependent diabetes in young people in the United Kingdom, have gathered new evidence which they believe reveals why teenagers experience badly controlled diabetes.

A survey among 90 teenagers by medical researchers in Dundee found that, on average, half the young patients did not take their insulin on over 100 days a year. Dr Ray Newton, who is in charge of diabetes services in Dundee, said this simple explanation reveals why controlling diabetes in adolescents is often so very difficult.

The medical teams were able to pinpoint the root cause of problems during the teen years through a unique method of monitoring the encashment of insulin prescriptions in Scotland. They found that young people with the most uncontrolled diabetes were also most likely to be the ones who failed to encash their insulin prescriptions. The authorities in Scotland, where 25 young people in every 100,000 under the age of 20 have insulin-dependent diabetes, now plan to take this work forward and find new strategies to help young people come to terms with their condition. These will include telephone helplines, and improved adolescent clinics which could become role models for every region.

Adolescent clinics

Many diabetes practitioners now recognize the importance of having a special clinic just for teenagers. They are often informal and specifically geared to young people, and they provide helpful advice as well as a chance to meet other young people of the same age with diabetes.

Most young people outgrow a children's clinic around the age of 15 or 16. The options then are to find a clinic for adolescents, use a hospital out-patient clinic or visit a private diabetes specialist or your own medical practitioner. But it is best for teenagers to have some contact with a clinic. If the problems of adolescence are not addressed, young people have a tendency to disappear from formal contact, feeling that they have outgrown the children's clinics and worried by what they see at the adult clinics. This loss of contact can have disastrous consequences for their future health, as the clinic needs to keep an eye on the first signs of any long-term complications such as eye or nerve disease.

Try and find a clinic which offers:

- health advice for young people
- friendly, helpful staff
- sessions in the evenings
- support groups and a telephone helpline
- the opportunity for your daughter to see a female doctor if she so wishes
- privacy during consultations
- a non-confrontational, non-threatening approach, using compromise and negotiation rather than imposing strict rules
- encouragement to teenagers on the road to becoming responsible for their lives
- a supportive atmosphere

At the clinic, teenagers can expect the following tests:

- eye tests to ensure that the tiny blood vessels at the back of the eye are healthy
- weighing and measuring to ensure that they are the right height and weight for their age
- blood tests to give them an idea of what blood glucose levels have been over the past couple of months
- blood pressure tests to ensure that the heart is pumping well
- tests on legs and feet to ensure that the nerves and circulation are all in order

The differences between boys and girls

Clare Williams, a medical researcher in the United Kingdom, has been looking at the differences between teenage boys and girls with diabetes, and attitudes towards taking responsibility for their own diabetes care. She interviewed ten girls and ten boys aged between 15 and 18, as well as their mothers, and found overwhelmingly that:

- girls took responsibility for their diabetes earlier
- girls felt more guilty if they neglected to have an insulin injection or ate something unsuitable
- boys liked the 'business' approach of a clinic whereas girls tended to seek out a more personal, sympathetic, one-to-one approach
- boys considered that they had good control, although their mothers often thought differently
- girls had more problems with diet than boys
- in general, boys exercised more than the girls

The reasons for poor diabetes control

Young people with diabetes fail to take their insulin regularly for a variety of reasons ranging from boredom, denial, manipulation or as a way to lose weight, to depression or simply because they 'could not be bothered'.

Poor diabetes control is common during the teenage years. Apart from a refusal to take insulin, the reasons include:

- poor eating habits
- heavy drinking
- a psychological problem involving the acceptance of diabetes

EATING DISORDERS

Ten per cent more teenagers with diabetes succumb to eating disorders than those without the disease. There are several reasons:

- Diabetes carries with it a natural preoccupation with food.
- There is an enormous feeling of guilt if a child eats ' the wrong thing'.

- Teenage girls with diabetes are often a little overweight, as insulin can encourage weight gain. The fear of having a hypo may prompt a young person to eat more snacks, adding to an existing weight problem.
- An eating disorder may be a cry for help – a channel for the teenager's confusion, anger or fear at the thought of a lifetime living with diabetes.

Bulimia and anorexia nervosa are the two most common eating disorders which affect young people with diabetes. Although most sufferers are girls, boys can also experience the disorders.

Bulimia may start as a psychological reaction to the pressures of diabetes, which can induce feelings of disgust, self-hatred and guilt. It may be used as a way of denying the diabetes as the young victim wrestles with the stresses and strains of coming to terms with this life-long condition and the demands of shouldering the huge responsibility that it involves.

Bulimia sufferers tend to binge on unsuitable foods and then vomit to get rid of the food. Teenage sufferers will store food in their rooms, or may disappear to the bathroom after eating a meal. There may well be huge swings in glucose levels. Anorexic victims are more often girls and this may coincide with pressures from their peers to lose weight or to be slim. Some teenagers become 'hooked' on the feel-good factor of being slim, and this may result in an obsessional avoidance of food.

Complementary therapies

Music therapy, autogenic training and reflexology may all help with eating disorders. A complementary therapist may give your child a chance to focus on the self and provide space to explore his problems.

Autogenics is rather like a Western meditation, and includes techniques of autosuggestion. It involves both the mind and the body, which is what makes it different from other forms of relaxation therapy. There are three basic parts: passive concentration, mental repetition of phrases associated with certain parts of the body (such as warmth and heaviness in the limbs), and the elimination of any arousing stimuli. It is a form of self-hypnosis that can modify the body's natural self-regulatory mechanisms. It also involves a set of six specific mental exercises which are repeated and used to help with stressful situations.

Teenagers and weight
One in 10 teenagers worry about their weight according to a MORI poll commissioned by the Royal College of Nursing in the United Kingdom and published in May 1996. And 86 per cent of the 4,295 young people aged between 11 and 16 who were interviewed said that they worried about they way they looked. The survey also compared teenagers from poor and well-off families, and found that more children from poorer backgrounds were concerned about being fat.

SEX

Sex education for young people with diabetes should be exactly the same as for any other teenagers. However, they will also have to learn some extra tips on keeping healthy in a sexually active relationship.

Every effort should be made to encourage open, frank discussion about sex. Teenagers with diabetes may be more acutely aware of their bodies – and what they may see as their bodies' failure – than other teenagers. They need to know that sex burns calories and energy, so that they not only need to take precautions against pregnancy but also against hypos! Girls with diabetes can take the contraceptive pill, as there are no extra risks, but they may notice a change in blood glucose levels, which will need monitoring.

DRINKING

Whether you like it or not teenagers will experiment with alcohol, but they should be aware that heavy drinking is one of the most common causes of ketoacidosis among young men with diabetes. It is also a major cause of hypos, so it is vital that they get the message that heavy drinking can be dangerous. In general, most young people drink more than the average – alcohol is a powerful aid to confidence.

As long as they follow certain guidelines, diabetics can join their friends for a drink, but they must know of the dangers of crossing the line. When they go out to a party, encourage them to have a snack beforehand, to dilute their alcohol with water or soft drink, and to eat later in the evening. Drinking on an empty stomach can be dangerous because of its immediate effect on blood glucose levels. They should use the following guidelines when they have a night out:

- Always eat when drinking.
- Alternate alcohol with a soft drink.
- Never drink on an empty stomach because this will automatically lower blood sugar levels and boost the influence of the alcohol, making your teenager less careful and possibly masking hypo signals.
- Symptoms of being drunk and having a hypo can be confused. Make sure your teenager wears an ID bracelet.
- Being drunk stops stores of glucose getting into the bloodstream, which is why heavy drinking is so dangerous for someone with diabetes.
- Check blood sugar levels before going to bed after a night out – it may be necessary to have an extra snack before sleep.

▨ DRUGS

Most young people are 'streetwise' about drugs such as ecstasy and cannabis by the age of 12 or 13, but the abuse of drugs will be dangerous for a teenager with diabetes. Cannabis has an acutely relaxing effect – it can raise blood glucose levels or mask the symptoms of a hypo. Ecstasy, which heightens the senses, can also bring on a hypo – it can cause dehydration and affect the kidneys. Any drug or solvent abuse can prompt your child to forget to take insulin, so parents should watch out for signs such as:

- needles, glue pots, or any other clues to drug taking in the bedroom
- bad glucose control
- extreme tiredness
- mood swings

Try and keep the lines of communication open, and get hold of as much information as possible about drug abuse so that you can have an informed conversation. As they have grown up with the idea of injecting substances to keep them alive, and with a more acute awareness of their body and their disease, young people with diabetes tend to be very sensible and well informed about drug taking.

HORMONES

Balancing diabetes and puberty is likely to be a difficult process for a year or so. Growth and sexual hormones act as counter-measures to insulin, so they can cause considerable problems for someone with diabetes until things start to settle down. Teenagers need to be reassured that even if control is poor for a while it really will not do them much harm in the long term. If they can accept it as a phase, and feel confident that control will be regained, then they will not feel under so much pressure to have consistently good blood sugar levels.

Many young women find that their blood sugar level falls and they crave sugar just before a period. If a teenage girl suffers from PMT, blood sugar levels may rise (as they can do with stress). Until her monthly cycle is established it will be very much a case of trial and error, but it will certainly help her if her mother is supporting her at this time.

▨ LETTING GO

During adolescence your role will be to keep yourself available when necessary to ensure a smooth ride to maturity. You will probably rely on ground rules established over the years – having a clear set of guidelines which you both understand will help most during the times of most confusion and chaos.

Letting go can be difficult. As the primary carer you will still want to know about your child's blood sugar levels, whether he has eaten, and when the last injection of insulin was. But drawing back is the only way to ensure that your child has the confidence, and eventually the maturity, to face the world. But it will not all be plain sailing.

Apart from the physical effects of adolescence, your child will also be facing new psychological challenges in the transition from child to adult. There will be occasions when the reality of diabetes will conflict with the teenager's image of who he would like to be. Adolescence is a time of experimentation and of discord, and when diabetes comes into the equation the result can, at times, be chaos. There will be times of recrimination – why me? – and rebellion at the pressures diabetes brings. It will be at times like this that your child will want to throw away the insulin and pretend, even for a day, that he no longer has diabetes.

Letting go means handing over the reins to your child. The process began with the first signs of independence as a toddler and continued in middle childhood, when the condition became more fully understood and he started to take responsibility for blood tests and injections. Now you face the final phase, during which you might still want to play a role. But be prepared to be accused of interfering or making a fuss. Your child may view all your advice about the snacks, getting enough sleep and so on as too embarrassing, and prefer to have nothing to do with it.

This will signal the time to take a step backwards and not press the issues. Above all remain calm, let things run their course and have confidence in your child, and in the fact that all the information you have provided over the years will finally pay off. It may sometimes seem as though you are on a cliff edge, but steel yourself, and you may well be pleasantly surprised at how well your child really is coping.

There will be times when you fear that your child is being less careful than you would be. You may feel frustrated, worried, even angry at no longer being in control. Talking about your worries and fears may help clear the air if your child is prepared to sit down and listen. But you must also be prepared to listen to the other side of the story and compromise on some of the issues.

Your priority during the teen years must be to ensure your child gains as much control over his life as possible. There will be highs and lows. As we have seen, these years are often fraught with difficult blood glucose levels because of puberty and the massive amounts of hormones which begin circulating in the body. Growth hormones can upset the best control, and this is bound to result in feelings of frustration for both of you. But even on the bad days you should remember that there will come a time when you will not ask whether your child has glucose tablets or a glucose drink in his college bag. When that day arrives you will know you have let go – successfully.

Conclusion

Living with diabetes is never going to be easy. But using holistic natural therapies will help you and your family find a new balance and calmness in your lives. Taking control of your child's health and trying different routes to optimum health is the underlying message of this book. The orthodox route is there to be followed, but there are other avenues to explore and, above all, to enjoy. I wish you good luck in finding the right route, and the right therapy, for you and your child.

Further reading

Barker, D J P, *Mothers, Babies and Disease in Later Life*, BMJ Publishing, UK, 1994

Day, John, *The Diabetes Handbook*, British Diabetic Association, 1986

Dunne, Desmond, *Yoga Made Easy*, Souvenir Press, UK, 1994

Estridge, Bonnie and Davies, Jo, *So Your Child Has Diabetes*, British Diabetic Association, 1993

Fontana, David and Slack, Ingrid, *Teaching Meditation to Children*, Element, UK, 1997

Govindji, Azmina and Myers, Jill, *Essential Diabetic Cookbook*, British Diabetic Association, 1994

Holford, Patrick, *Optimum Nutrition Workbook*, ION Press, UK, 1988

Hornsbury, W Guyton, *Fitness Book for People with Diabetes*, American Diabetes Association, 1994

Horrobin, David (ed), *Treatment for Diabetic Neuropathy: A New Approach*, Churchill Livingstone, UK/USA, 1992

Kirsta, Alixa, *Book of Stress Survival*, Unwin, UK, 1986

Lockie, Andrew, *Family Guide to Homoeopathy*, Hamish Hamilton, UK, 1990

Loring, Gloria, *Parenting a Diabetic Child*, Lowell House, USA, 1993

Murray, Michael and Pizzorno, Joseph, *Encylopaedia of Natural Medicine*, Optima, UK, 1994

Nagarathna, R, Nagendra, H R and Monro, Robin, *Yoga for Common Ailments*, Gaia Books, UK, 1990

Pietroni, Patrick (ed), *Reader's Digest Family Guide to Alternative Medicine*, Reader's Digest Association, UK, 1991

Shillitoe, Richard, *Counselling People with Diabetes*, British Psychological Society, UK, 1994 van Straten, Michael, *Complete Natural Health Consultant*, Ebury Press, UK, 1986

Weller, Cheryl (ed), *Learning to Live Well with Diabetes*, DCI Publishing, USA, 1991

Wildwood, Christine, *Aromatherapy: Massage with Essential Oils*, Element, UK, 1991

Useful addresses

INTERNATIONAL

**International Diabetes
Federation**
40 rue Washington
B – 1050 Brussels, Belgium
Tel: 322 647 4414
Fax: 322 640 8565

**International Diabetic Athletes
Association**
6829 North 12th Street
Suite 205
Phoenix, AZ 85014, USA
Tel: 602 230 8155

**International Federation of
Practitioners of Natural
Therapeutics**
10 Copse Close
Sheet, Petersfield
Hampshire GU31 4DL, UK
Tel: 01730 266790
Fax: 01730 260058

International Society of
Professional Aromatherapists
ISPA House
82 Ashby Road
Hinckley
Leics
LE10 1LW, UK

**Juvenile Diabetes Foundation
International**
The Diabetes Research
Foundation
432 Park Avenue South
New York
NY 10016 8013, USA
Tel: 212 889 7575/800 223 1138

World Health Organization
Division of Noncommunicable
Diseases
1211 Geneva 27
Switzerland
Tel: 4122 791 3472
Fax: 4122 791 0746

■ AUSTRALASIA

Australian Natural Therapists Association
PO Box 308
Melrose Park
South Australia 5039
Tel: 618 297 9533
Fax: 618 297 0003

Australian Traditional Medicine Society
PO Box 442 *or*
Suite 3, First Floor
120 Blaxland Road
Ryde
New South Wales 2112
Australia
Tel: 612 808 2825
Fax: 612 809 7570

Diabetes Australia
AVA House
5/7 Phipps Place
Deakin
ACT 2600, Australia
Tel: 616 285 3277
Fax: 616 285 2881

Diabetes New Zealand Inc
1 Coquet Street
PO Box 54
Oamaru, 8915
South Island
New Zealand
Tel: 643 434 8110
Fax: 643 434 5281

New Zealand Natural Health Practitioners Accreditation Board
PO Box 37-491
Auckland, New Zealand
Tel: 9 625 9966
Supported by 15 therapy organizations

■ NORTH AMERICA

American Academy of Medical Preventics
6151 West Century Boulevard
Suite 1114
Los Angeles
California 90045, USA
Tel: 213 645 5350

American Association of Naturopathic Physicians
2800 East Madison Street
Suite 200
Seattle
Washington 98112, USA
or
PO Box 20386
Seattle
Washington 98102, USA
Tel: 206 323 7610
Fax: 206 323 7612

American Diabetes Association
1660 Duke Street
Alexandria
VA 22314, USA
Tel: 703 549 1500
Fax: 703 836 7439

American Dietetic Association
216 West Jackson Boulevard
Suite 800
Chicago IL 60606, USA
Tel: 312 899 0040
Fax: 800 877 1600

**American Holistic Medical
Association**
6728 Old Mclean
Village Drive
Mclean
VA 22101, USA
Tel: 703556 9222

Canadian Diabetes Association
15 Toronto Street, Suite 1001
Toronto
Ontario M5C 2E3, Canada
Tel: 416 363 3373
Fax: 416 363 3393

**Canadian Holistic Medical
Association**
700 Bay Street
PO Box 101, Suite 604
Toronto
Ontario M5G 1Z6, Canada
Tel: 416 599 0447

**L'Association du Diabete du
Quebec**
5635 Sherbrooke Estate
Montreal
Quebec H1N 1A3, Canada
Tel: 514 259 3422
Fax: 514 259 9286

■ SOUTH AFRICA

**South African Diabetes
Association**
PO Box 3943
Cape Town 8000
South Africa
Tel: 2721 461 3715
Fax: 2721 462 2008

**South African Homoeopaths,
Chiropractors & Allied
Professions Board**
PO Box 17055
0027 Groenkloof
South Africa
Tel: 1246 6455

■ UNITED KINGDOM & EIRE

Association of Stress Therapists
5 Springfield Road
Palm Bay
Clintonville
Kent
CT9 3EA

British Complementary Medicine Association
St Charles Hospital
Exmoor Street
London W10 6DZ
Tel: 0181 964 1205
Fax: 0181 964 1207

British Diabetic Association
10 Queen Anne Street
London
W1M 0BD

British Holistic Medical Association
Trust House
Royal Shrewsbury Hospital
(South)
Shrewsbury
Shropshire SY3 8XF
Tel: 01743 261155
Fax: 01743 3536373

British Homoeopathic Association
27A Devonshire Street
London
W1N 1RJ

British Hypnotherapy Association
67 Upper Berkeley Street
London
W1H 7DH

British Nutrition Foundation
High Holborn House
52–4 High Holborn
London WC1V 6RQ

Council for Complementary & Alternative Medicine
179 Gloucester Place
London NW1 6DX
Tel: 0171 724 9103
Fax: 0171 724 5330

General Council and Register of Naturopaths
Goswell House
2 Goswell Road
Street
Somerset
BA16 0JG

Health Education Authority
Hamilton House
Mabledon Place
London WC1H 9TX
Tel: 0171 383 3833
Fax: 0171 387 0550

Institute for Complementary Medicine
PO Box 194
London SE16 1QZ
Tel: 0171 237 5165
Fax: 0171 237 5175

Institute for Optimum Nutrition
13 Blades Court
Deodor Road
London
SW15 2NU

Irish Diabetic Association
76 Lower Gardiner Street
Dublin 1, Eire
Tel/fax: 353 136 3022

Juvenile Diabetes Federation (UK)
25 Gosfield Street
London
W1P 8EB

Massage Training Institute
24 Highbury Road
London
N5 2DQ

N H Eastwood and Son
118 East Barnet Road
Barnet
Herts
EN4 8RE

UK Council for Psychotherapy
167–9 Great Portland Street
London
W1N 5FB

Yoga Biomedical Trust
PO Box 140
Cambridge
CB4 3SY

Index

Note: where more than one reference is given, main references are indicated in **bold**